中医外宣翻译教程

主编 高 芸

副主编 马白菊 叶丽珍 张忆萍

戴 乐 张忆萍 周澄雷

审校 薛玲玲 王佳鑫

U0295109

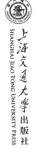

上海交通大学出版社

SHANGHAI JIAO TONG UNIVERSITY PRESS

内容提要

本教材聚焦中医外宣翻译和应用翻译的主要文本类型，覆盖中医药政府文书、中医药新闻、中医药科研论文、中医药科普读物、中成药说明书、中医药企事业网上简介、中医药公示语等。通过提供丰富的中医药汉英平行文本语料，引导学生从文本功能出发，基于语料对比分析，从篇章、段落和句子等层次进行翻译调整，从而产生符合行业规范、能被西方读者接受的译文。本教材最后一章提供了中医药真实翻译项目教学案例，帮助学生运用翻译技术，熟悉实际翻译项目操作流程，掌握各个角色所需要的技能。本教材适用于中医外语或翻译硕士生的翻译教学，也可供中医外语专业本科生翻译教学选用。

图书在版编目(CIP)数据

中医外宣翻译教程 / 高芸主编. -- 上海 ： 上海交通大学出版社，2025. 1. -- ISBN 978-7-313-31761-2

Ⅰ. R2

中国国家版本馆 CIP 数据核字第 2024H7X658 号

中医外宣翻译教程

ZHONGYI WAIXUAN FANYI JIAOCHENG

主　　编：高　芸

出版发行：上海交通大学出版社　　　　　地　　址：上海市番禺路 951 号

邮政编码：200030　　　　　　　　　　　电　　话：021 - 64071208

印　　制：苏州市古得堡数码印刷有限公司　经　　销：全国新华书店

开　　本：787 mm×1092 mm　1/16

字　　数：267 千字

版　　次：2025 年 1 月第 1 版　　　　　　印　　次：2025 年 1 月第 1 次印刷

书　　号：ISBN 978 - 7 - 313 - 31761 - 2

定　　价：68.00 元

印　　张：15

前　　言

　　2022年10月，习近平总书记在二十大报告中指出："加快构建中国话语和中国叙事体系，讲好中国故事、传播好中国声音，展现可信、可爱、可敬的中国形象。"作为一种重要的跨文化实践，对外翻译在中国形象构建中的作用不容忽视。随着国家实施文化外译战略，对外翻译"不仅要研究传统的以语言作为表达媒介的翻译，更要关注作为国家形象建构之载体的跨文化的翻译和阐述"（王宁，2018：6）。中医药外宣翻译对讲好中医药文化故事，推动中医药文化走出去，树立正面、全面的中国文化形象起着重要的作用。中医药翻译硕士作为服务于社会、经济、文化领域的专业翻译人才，为担负起中医文化海外传播的责任，应具备中国文化自觉和文化自信，具有全球视野与国际化服务能力（余环、邓凌云，2019：40），能够用海外读者所能听懂、读懂的语言对外讲好中医文化故事，诠释新时代语境下的中医文化形象（高芸，2020：65）。一个优秀的中医药译者不仅需要精通两种语言，还要了解与这两种不同语言密不可分的两种不同的文化，具备"融通中外的叙事能力"（任文，2018：95），要能够以目标语读者为取向，迎合目标语读者的信息需求、知识文化背景、思维方式和阅读习惯，借鉴目标语同类文本规范，根据翻译任务和具体情境对翻译策略做出灵活、合理的选择，产出符合行业规范、能被读者所接受的译文。

　　为了满足新时代对中医药翻译硕士生翻译能力的要求，本教材旨在帮助学生领会、掌握中医药外宣翻译主要文本类型的预期功能和翻译特征，并提升根据文本功能和行业规范灵活运用翻译策略的能力。同时，促进学生政治认同、家国情怀、文化素养、道德修养的培养。前一个目标与学习翻译知识和技能相关，称为显性目标；后一个目标与思政育人有关，称为隐性目标，需要教师有意识地引领学生思考。本教材拟通过融合显性和隐性教学目标，促进具有国际视野与家国情怀的中医药翻译人才的培养。本教材单元教学目标分解如下表所示。

《中医外宣翻译教程》教学目标分解

单元	主题	知识目标	能力目标	价值目标
一	中医药外宣翻译理论与教学	中医药外宣翻译定义、特征、文本类型等	中医药外宣翻译多元化翻译意识	政治认同、文化自信等
二	中医药政府文书英译	政府文书文本功能与翻译特点	中医药政府文书全译策略能力	政治认同、文化自信等
三	中医药新闻译写	新闻文本功能与翻译特点	中医药新闻编译策略能力	政治认同、文化自信等
四	中医药科研论文译写	科研论文功能与翻译特点	中医药科研论文译写策略能力	学术诚信、伦理道德等
五	中医药科普读物英译	科普读物文本功能与翻译特点	中医药科普读物翻译策略能力	家国情怀、敬业精神等
六	中成药说明书英译	说明书文本功能与翻译特点	中成药说明书改译策略能力	家国情怀、文化素养等
七	中医药企事业单位网页简介英译	网页简介文本功能与翻译特点	中医药网上简介改译策略能力	家国情怀、文化素养等
八	中医药公示语英译	公示语文本功能与翻译特点	中医药公示语改译策略能力	家国情怀、文化素养等
九	中医药外宣翻译工作坊	翻译技术与实际翻译项目操作流程	操作流程中各个角色的技能	职业规范、职业素养等

为实现以上教学目标,本教程覆盖中医药翻译多种文本类型,并根据文本功能进行编排:第二章至五章涉及的文本以实现信息功能为主,包括中医药政府文书、新闻、科研论文和科普读物四种文本类型;第六、七、八章涉及的文本主要发挥感染功能,包括中成药说明书、中医药企事业单位网页简介和公示语三种文本类型。该编排方法有利于体现不同文本类型在翻译方法和策略上的差异,并引导学生从文本预期功能出发,根据英译规范,从文本层面对原文进行适度的改译、节译和编译,从而提升译文的质量和传播效果。需要说明的是,虽然中医典籍英译也重在信息表达,但对译者的语言和翻译能力要求更高,需进行专门教学,故本教材没有涉及。

此外,本教材围绕政治认同、家国情怀、文化素养、道德修养等方面,选取译论、译作、译者、译例、行业等角度,深入挖掘中医药翻译德育资源。译论资源包括中医传统译论和西方翻译理论。中医传统译论深受中国传统文化的影响,蕴含丰富的文化资源,有利于提升学生对中医文化的自我认知与认同,以及对中医文化价值的充分肯定与积极践行。如在术语翻译教学中引入"语言国情学"理论,可以说明"阴阳"的音译形式"yin and yang"能准确完整地揭示阴阳主旨内涵,因此目前已普遍为海内外学者所接受并已收入《韦氏大词典》(*Webster's Dictionary*)(李照国,2017:6)。同时,引进德国功能翻译学派等西方翻译理论,有助于学生拓展国际视野,通过中西方翻译理论对比分析,提升对本国理论的认知能力。在译作资源方面,将中西方译作融入教材,有助于提升学生文化自信,加深对中西方文明交流互鉴和中西医双向融合的理解。译者资源包括中西方著名译者,如罗希文、谢竹藩、李照国等国内中医药翻译家,以及魏迺杰(Nigel Wiseman)、文树德(Paul U. Unschuld)、马万里(Giovanni Maciocia)等在国际上对中医药翻译和传播作出突出贡献的海外译者。中国翻译家的爱国主义情怀和无私奉献精神,以及西方知名译者的精益求精的科研精神,都将有助于学生家国情怀和价值观的培养。在译例资源方面,通过选择中医大家的故事,引导学生深刻理解医者仁心、大医精诚等核心精神,以及讲仁爱、重民本、守诚信、崇正义等中华优秀传统文化中的思想精华。《中国的中医药》等政府文书是将知识传授与价值引领相结合的理想学习资源。行业资源以翻译职业素养要求为主,通过组织实施中医药翻译项目,帮助学生形成爱岗敬业、扎实严谨、勇于开拓、开放合作的职业规范和素养。

全书共九章。第一章概述中医药外宣翻译理论与教学,介绍了中医药外宣翻译基本概念与主要特征、德国功能学派翻译理论在中医药外宣翻译理论与教学中的应用,为后面章节提供理论支撑。第二章至第八章为中医药外宣翻译主要文本类型英译,其中第二章至第七章从语料导入入手,提供汉英中医药平行文本,然后按照篇章—段落—词语的顺序展开分析。教师引导学生对语料库提供的典型、真实、丰富的译例进行观察、分析和思考,帮助学生通过批判性阅读,了解中医药外宣翻译文本类型的主要功能与语篇特征,进而掌握按照从语篇到段落,再到句子和词语的顺序,自上而下对原文进行适应性变通的翻译策略。第八章为中医药公示语英译,因该文本多为句子,所以章节编排方式有所不同。第九章为中医药真实翻译项目教学案例,旨在帮助学生运用翻译技术,熟悉实际翻译项目操作流程,掌握各个角色所需要的技能。教程的每个章节都提供了翻译练习与任务。翻译练习旨在帮助学生掌握基本翻译策略与技能,为完成翻译任务做准备;翻译任务要求学生采取小组合作学习的形式,根据文本功能、翻译目的、目标受众等因素,灵活运用策略进行翻译,并思考翻译内容所蕴含的思政元素。每项任务根据其复杂程度,给予1~2周的时间完成,最后每个小组汇报本组的翻译任务实施情况,教师进行最后的总结和点评。

本教材将《中医外宣翻译理论与教学实践》①一书中阐述的翻译理论应用到教学实践,并对该书中的教学案例部分进行了扩充和完善,从而适用于中医外语或翻译硕士生的翻译教学。本书可作为"中医药外宣翻译"或"中医药应用翻译"课程的配套教材使用,也可供中医药外语专业本科生翻译教学选用。

本教材第一章、第四章、第五章、第六章和第七章由高芸编写,第二章由马白菊编写,第三章由叶丽珍编写,第八章由张忆萍编写,第九章由周澄雷编写,薛玲玲、戴乐和王佳鑫负责全书的校对。本教材若有不妥之处,敬请批评指正。

---

① 高芸.中医外宣翻译理论与教学实践[M].上海:上海交通大学出版社,2023.

目　　录

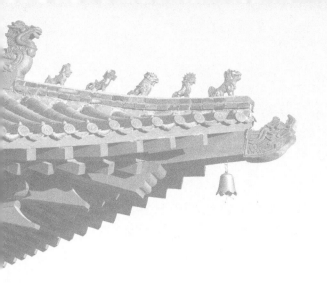

第一章
中医药外宣翻译
理论与教学

本章在介绍中医药外宣翻译概念和主要文本类型的基础上，厘清中医药外宣翻译不同于传统中医药翻译的特征，并基于德国功能学派翻译理论，构建中医药外宣翻译教学模式，为第二章至第八章提供理论基础。

第一节　中医药外宣翻译理论概述

一、中医药外宣翻译定义和资料

外宣翻译（C-E Translation for China's Global Communication）是对国际交流与传播在翻译方面活动的统称，是在当前全球化背景下，以让世界了解中国为目的、以汉语为信息源、以英语等外国语为信息载体、以各种媒体为渠道、以外国民众（包括境内的各类外籍人士）为对象的交际活动（张健，2013a：19）。中医药外宣翻译，顾名思义，就是将有关中医药的信息通过各种途径对外传播，使外国人了解中医、接受中医，从而让中医药走向世界（罗海燕、邓海静，2017：567）。

外宣翻译资料有广义和狭义之分。广义的外宣翻译包括除文学翻译之外的所有应用文体的翻译。狭义的外宣翻译主要包括五类文本的翻译：政治文献资料翻译、新闻文本翻译、公示语翻译、信息资料翻译以及汉语典籍翻译（卢小军，2015：10）。本教材采用广义的外宣翻译资料概念，即和中医药相关的所有应用文本，如典籍文献、政府文书、新闻文本、科研论文、医院公示语、宣传资料、说明书、商务广告等。随着世界经济的发展和商业化程度的进一步提高，应用翻译所占比例将有增无减（李长栓,2004:20),采取广义的外宣翻译资料概念有助于更好地满足市场对应用型中医药翻译人才的巨大需求。

二、中医药外宣翻译特征

中医药外宣翻译和传统中医药翻译相比,除了文本类型更为广泛,在翻译方向、翻译目的、目标受众、翻译策略等方面的特征非常鲜明,值得学习者深入了解。

1. 中医药外宣翻译属于译出行为

译出与译入是方向相反的翻译行为,如中医典籍翻译对于西方译者而言是译入行为,而对于中国译者而言是译出行为。随着"文化走出去"和"一带一路"倡议的实施,中医药文化外译正在成为翻译的重要内容。中医药外宣翻译通过中医药典籍、新闻文本、政府文书等文本种类的英译,正成为讲述中医故事、传播中医药文化、展示中医药形象的重要路径。同时,近年来我国逐步加快中医药国际化进程,越来越多的中医药产品和服务产业跨出国门,争取国际市场的承认和认可,由此产生了大量中医药应用翻译译出任务,如企事业单位宣传资料、中药说明书、外贸函电等。谢天振教授(2019:95-102)指出,译出与译入不仅方向不同,两者在翻译标准和策略上也存在实质性差异。在当今西方文化仍占据强势地位的世界文化格局下,为增强译文在国外的接受度,译介者不仅须译得忠实、准确、流畅,更须关注制约和影响翻译活动成败得失的相关因素,如目标读者的阅读习惯、审美情趣,目的语国家的意识形态、诗学观念等。

2. 中医药外宣翻译注重目的性和传播效果

中医药外宣翻译具有明确的目的性,即推动中医药文化在海外广泛传播,深化世界对中医药文化的了解,树立正向、全面的中医药文化形象,从而助推中国良好国际形象的树立。为此,中医药外宣翻译十分注重传播效果,力图使"信息到达目的地后引起的各种反应"(张健,2008:24)和预期一致。张健教授指出:"翻译是一个很专业的领域,判断一个译者是否合格、优秀,不能仅仅局限于语言文字转换的层面上,标尺之一是他翻译的作品是否符合行业规范,是否被读者所接受,是否达到预期目的,能否在跨文化语境中得以有效传播并产生应有的影响。否则,语言文字转换得再好也不能算是成功的翻译。"(张健,2013b:VII)换言之,中医药外宣翻译的传播效果是决定翻译成功与否的关键所在,如果传播出去的信息不被国外受众接受或者效果不佳,中医药外宣翻译就失去了传播意义。由于社会制度、文化背景和意识形态的不同,国内外话语体系存在一定的差异。在全球化背景下,为加强中医药外宣翻译的传播效果,让国际社会更易于理解和接受中医药文化的核心概念与表述,译者要有说"全球话"的思维,使其对接国外惯用的话语体系、表达方式,按照目标受众的信息需求、阅读习惯进行信息的转换,突出翻译的交际性特征,帮助他们明确无误地理解和获得译文所传递的信息要旨。

3. 中医药外宣翻译强调受众内外有别

受众是翻译行为关注的焦点,原因很简单:现实生活中,翻译的根本在于影响受众,翻译目的的实现有赖于受众对译者和翻译话语的认同、信奉和在此基础上改变态度或采取行动(陈小慰,2012:94)。为此,译者需要具备受众意识,即在翻译过程中以关注、认识和了解目标受众为指导,进行自己的实践活动的意识(卢小军,2015:97)。外宣翻译十分强调国内外受众的不同。国内资深记者和翻译家基于多年翻译经验和跨文化交流实践,总结出"外宣三贴近"原则对中医药外宣翻译具有指导意义,即为使外宣取得预期效果,中国的国际交际活动必须贴近中国实际发展阶段,交际活动内容必须贴近目标受众想了解中国的信息需求,外宣翻译文本必须贴近目标语文化的惯例和规范(黄友义,2004:27-28)。

国内外受众由于生活在不同的地理、社会、语言和文化环境中,他们对信息内容的兴趣、需求各不相同。外宣翻译首先要贴近目标受众想了解中国的信息需求。在了解外国受众需求的时候,必须明确目标受众是谁,他们的知识背景如何。国务院新闻办公室原主任赵启正认为,一定要把外国的受众对中国的理解假设为一个外国中学毕业生,万万不能假设为一个专家,否则会把我们的书写得太深、太涩,这样写成中文都未必能吸引很多中国读者,更不用说翻译成外文面向外国读者了(贾树枚,2018:163)。其次,贴近外国受众的思维习惯。对外宣传不只是语言和文字的翻译,而且是文化和思想的翻译。为达到预期的对外传播效果,外宣翻译需从目标受众的角度出发,充分研究国外受众的文化惯例和规范,提供给他们内容和形式都十分地道的外文翻译。如果在对外宣传中不注意"内外有别",直接套用对内宣传的内容和形式,轻则贻笑大方,重则可能影响甚至有损国家形象。中医药翻译工作者只有注重受众内外有别,跨越时间差、地域差、语言差和文化差,从目标受众的角度出发,才能更好地对外传播中医药知识与文化。

4. 中医药外宣翻译采取多元化翻译策略

翻译界长久以来以"信、达、雅"作为翻译的基准,即注重并追求"完整准确""忠实原文""语言优美"等。与此相类似的表达还有"形似神似""案本求信""译作如著"等,都对传统翻译实践起着一定的指导作用。但是,传统的翻译标准已不能完全适应新时代语境对外宣翻译的要求。翻译从来不是一种"机械性的工作",而是一种"创造性的工作"(爱泼斯坦、林戊荪、沈苏儒,2000:3)。外宣翻译资深专家段连城

(2004：176－177)曾最早提出,在翻译一般性对外宣传材料(非官方文件)时,应允许译者对材料的中文原稿进行适当加工。加工策略包括增加背景信息,帮助目标读者充分了解翻译内涵;避免陈词滥调和空洞的字面翻译,采用符合目标受众文化规范的恰当的语言,提供字面翻译背后的信息;根据目标读者文化的规范和惯例重新调整译文的文本布局,例如句子排序,甚至是段落排序。张健(2013a：20)指出外宣译者必须有意识地根据译文读者的特殊要求,采用编译、改写等"变通"手法,改变源语文本的内容和结构,乃至风格,以方便目的语读者接受,使目的语文本更通顺、更清楚、更直接,更好地实现交际目的。曾剑平(2018：243)提出在语篇翻译中,需从平行文本角度出发,以翻译功能理论、文本类型理论和变译理论为指导,针对不同的外宣翻译文本,采用全译、改译、编译等翻译策略,以符合译文读者的思维方式和目的语的行文习惯。

中医药外宣翻译采取多元化的翻译策略是提升译文传播力的必然要求,多元化的翻译策略不仅包括全译,还包括节译、改译、编译、译写等。全译通常是逐段将全文译完,不得故意遗漏(方梦之、毛忠明,2018：44),许多中医典籍文献、歌赋均采取全译。但对中医药外宣翻译而言,全译不是主要的翻译方式,节译、改译、编译、译写等形式更加普遍。节译指有选择地翻译全文的一部分或大部分,译者选择全文的主要信息,删去枝节,或选择读者感兴趣的信息(同上注),如美国学者爱尔萨·威斯(Ilza Veith)女士为了从医史的角度帮助西方了解《黄帝内经·素问》的概貌,翻译了这部中医典籍的前34章。改译是为达到预期目的,在翻译时对原文内容进行一定程度的改变,或对小到词语,大到语段等形式进行重大调整,以适应译入语国家或读者的政治语境、文化背景或技术规范(方梦之、毛忠明,2018：49),如中医药应用文本的改译主要出于对尽可能实现文本的信息、感染功能以及预期交际目的,符合文本规范的综合考虑。编译是译者在节译的基础上,为更适合译入语读者的阅读口味和习惯,在不改变原文信息的前提下所做的文字处理(方梦之、毛忠明,2018：51),如中医药新闻英译的编译一方面可以给海外读者带去形式熟悉且易于理解的新闻,另一方面也可以服务于主流意识形态,提升国家形象。

第二节　德国功能学派翻译理论与应用

国内外近几十年的翻译研究重点从词语、句子等微观层面向语篇、文本等宏观层面转向,注重翻译理论对语言具体应用的指导作用。其中,由德国功能学派翻译理论的代表人物卡塔琳娜·莱斯(Katharina Reiss)、汉斯·J. 费米尔(Hans J. Vermeer)、克里斯蒂安妮·诺德(Christiane Nord)等学者提出并加以完善的功能翻译理论便是较有影响的理论之一。该理论对于中医药外宣翻译也具有理论研究与教学应用上的价值。

一、德国功能学派文本类型理论与应用

1. 德国功能学派文本类型理论

德国功能主义翻译理论代表人物莱斯在《翻译批评:潜力与制约》一书中首次引入了功能语言理论,并提出了文本类型与语言功能及翻译策略的关系,强调文本层面的对等,并将语言功能与文本类型及翻译策略联系起来。莱斯(Reiss,1977/1989)根据文本的主要功能,将所有文本主要分为三种类型:信息型(informative)、表情型(expressive)和操作型(operative)。她指出,划分文本类型的意义在于文本类型确定总的翻译方法策略(Reiss,1981/2000),三种文本类型的语言功能及其与翻译方法的联系如表1-1所示。之后,德国功能主义翻译理论另一名代表人物诺德将操作型改称为感染型(appellative)。这个称呼在译界接受度更广,故下文采用后者称呼。莱斯阐述的文本主要功能决定翻译方法的理论,对于分析翻译问题、制定翻译策略具有现实指导意义,"超越了纯语言的层面、超越了纸上的文字及其意义,把视野拓宽到翻译的交际目的"(Munday,2001:76)。

表1-1　文本类型的功能特点及其与翻译方法的联系(Munday,2001:74)

文本类型	信息型	表情型	操作型
语言功能	表现事物与事实	表达情感与态度	感染文本接受者
语言特点	逻辑的	审美的	对话的
文本焦点	侧重内容	侧重形式	侧重感染作用
译文目的	表达其内容	表现其形式	引出所期望的反应
翻译方法	平实的语言、简洁明了	仿效、忠实原作	编译、等效

2. 中医药外宣翻译文本类型划分与建库

中医药外宣翻译文本按照传递的主要功能可分为三大类:信息型文本,包括中医典籍文献、学术论文与报告、政府文书、教科书、新闻文本等;表情型文本,仅限于中医药文学作品;感染型文本,包括中医药说明书、企事业单位宣传资料、医院公示语、

广告等。本书采用广义的中医药外宣翻译资料定义,研究除文学作品之外的所有中医药应用文本,这些文本主要发挥信息和感染两种功能。实际上,由于大多数中医药外宣翻译文本兼具信息与感染功能,很难绝对将某一种文本归为信息型或感染型。即使如此,每一种文本预期发挥的功能总是有主有次的,通过归类文本类型,译者可以根据文本主要功能采取适当的翻译策略(张美芳,2013:6)。以中医典籍为例,有学者将其归为表情型文本。李照国教授早在1997年就提出"薄文重医、依实出华"的中医药翻译原则,即译文要摆脱中医语言中文学色彩的影响,实事求是、客观准确(李照国,1997:16)。因此,将中医典籍文献归为信息型文本较为合适。中医典籍英译注重原文的形式还是内容,很大程度上取决于不同历史文化语境下的翻译目的和目标读者。又如,中成药说明书英译的功能之一是提供给海外消费者药品信息,但同时具有激发海外消费者的购买欲、推动他们最终采取购买该药品行动的重要功能。为突出说明书的宣传作用,本书将其归为感染型文本。

为选取适当的翻译策略,译者不仅要分析每种文本功能的普遍性,还要研究同类型文本的特殊性(方梦之,2017:5),可以按照语境,从语场(指语言发生的环境,交际的主题也算在内,它可以反映出语言使用者的目的)、语旨(指交际参与者所扮演的角色以及他们之间的关系)、语式(指语言交际的媒介或渠道,可以是专业性的或非专业性的,需要选用不同的言语风格)三个语域变量入手进一步细分。例如,中医药公司、高校和中医医院的网页简介具有不同的交际目的,公司网页简介英译对感染力和亲和力的要求明显高于其他两种文本,因此译者在翻译不同类型企事业单位宣传资料时须调整翻译策略;再如,中医典籍英译的目标受众在不同的社会历史文化背景下有所不同,译者根据语旨不同,选择归化或异化翻译策略可满足目标受众的信息需求差异,从而更好地实现译文的预期功能;而对于中医药宣传片而言,字幕须随画面出现,停留的时间也有限,所以译者必须采取照顾时空的翻译策略,压缩信息,用词简明,让观众一目了然。

平行文本,也称平行语篇,在翻译研究和教学领域广泛使用,通常指不同语言中话语单位的源语形态因交际功能相近或相似而具有对比参照价值。对各自原生性语篇展开比较,可以从根本上审视两种语言对同一或类似交际情景下的话语习惯和行为方式,给译者提供有关体裁、文体常规、表达形式、搭配、习惯用语、语域等方面的信息,并在翻译时加以借鉴,有效提高译文的可读性和影响力(陈小慰,2017:1-2)。国际著名词典学家哈特曼(Hartmann,1980:37-40)把平行文本分为三类:A类为形式上非常一致的译文及原文,在语义上对等,在形式上尽可能多地保留原文的某些特色;B类为形式上不完全一致,但功能对等的译文及原文,又称为改写对应语料,即同一信息用两种不同的语言来表达所得到的对应语料;C 类为语域对应语料,这类对应语料不再具有语义上的对应性,而只是在语篇的题材风格、使用场合、使用对象等方面具有某种一致性。本教材用于文本分析的中医药外宣翻译平行文本均为 C 类,指具有类似或相同体裁,实施相同功能,而不具有语义对应性的源语(汉语)文本和目标(英语)文本。构建中医药外宣翻译平行文本语料库要求收集的各类文本具有代表性和可比性,并且尽量平行度高。

二、德国功能学派文本分析模式与应用

1. 德国功能学派文本分析模式

翻译是将源语文本转换成译语文本的过程,因此翻译离不开文本分析(胡珍铭、王湘玲,2018:79)。诺德从文本功能的视角提出以翻译为导向的文本分析模式,这种模式更加关注原文的特色(杰里米·芒迪,2014:123),可用于对原文中一系列复杂且具有内在相关性的超文本因素及文本内因素进行分析。诺德提出文本是由语言和非语言手段共同实现的动态交际过程,文本分析不仅要分析文本本身,还要分析翻译作为一种社会行为所受到的社会制约性因素。文本内因素包括主题、内容、前提、构成、非语言因素(插图、斜体等)、句型结构、词汇、超音段特征等;超文本因素包括文本发送者及其意图、接受者及其期望、文本媒介、文本交际场所和时间、动机等。文本分析过程中,文本内因素和超文本因素存在着密切关系,两者相互影响、相互制约(Nord,2005:43-143)。文本接受的情境、社会背景、接受者的知识背景以及交际需求共同决定了读者对文本的期待与接受度,并最终决定文本功能。在具体翻译过程中,译者首先要对实现源文功能的各种文本内因素、超文本因素与连贯机制有着清晰的解读,然后将之与目的文本的特定文化情境、功能以及语内连贯机制进行对比,从而确定如何对原文进行适应性变通(同上)。

超文本概念及研究方法来自法籍文学理论家杰哈·简奈特(Gérard Genette)。简奈特(1997:4)认为,研究各种超文本成分,就是研究其各种特征,例如时间的、空间的、具体的、时效的、功能的。根据简奈特所建立的超文本概念框架,某一个超文本成分包括其所处的情景(where)、出现和消失的时间(when)、存在的形式(how)、信息发送者与接收者(from whom to whom)及信息的预定功能(to do what)等等(转引自张美芳,2011:51)。如今,超文本范畴已从纯文学作品拓宽到非文学作品,超文本的定义扩大到文本产生的政治体制、文化环境、经济条件、审查制度等大环境因素,超文本的作用也从对读者施加影响拓展到对文本翻译策略的规范、制约作用。当代国

际著名翻译理论家安德烈·勒弗唯尔(Andre Lefevere)将翻译研究与权力、意识形态、赞助人和诗学结合起来,认为意识形态主要从政治、经济和社会地位方面来限制和引导译者的创作,而诗学形态则是译者进行创作时所处的文化体系的重要组成部分。译者经常不由自主地对原作进行适当的调整,使之符合占统治地位的意识形态和诗学形态(Lefevere,1992:7-8)。赞助人可以是宗教集团、政府部门、出版社、大众传媒机构等,也可以是个人势力。它是主流意识形态的代言人,往往集意识形态、经济和社会地位的影响力于一身。在实际的翻译中,最重要的往往不是译者能否创造出和原文相似的译文,而是译者能否在迎合赞助人的期望、尊重意识形态规范的同时,完成翻译使命(同上注:17)。

诺德明确提出"从上至下"的文本分析和翻译路径。她认为,传统的翻译方法从微观层面的词语分析入手,上升到宏观层面的语篇分析,这种"从下至上"的顺序会过于注重源语文本的结构,而忽略译文的预期交际功能,从而不可避免地导致一系列语用、文化以及语言方面的翻译问题。为解决翻译问题,译者需要首先明确译文预期发挥的交际功能是文献型(展示原文作者与接收者之间进行文化交流的文献,如文学翻译)还是工具型(在目标语文化的交际行为中充当独立的信息传递工具,以实现新的交际目的而不让读者感到陌生,如应用文体翻译),然后在此基础上决定翻译风格。文献型翻译应以源语文化为导向,而工具型翻译则以目标语文化为导向,有关文本的问题可以在较低的语言层面得以解决(Nord,2001:39)。

2. 中医药外宣翻译文本分析

诺德的文本分析模式对于实施中医药外宣翻译文本分析具有指导意义。为推动中医药文化走出去,中医药翻译研究被置于更为广阔的社会历史与文化语境之中,不仅需要关注翻译的内部研究,即从文本到文本的转换过程,还要关注翻译的外部研究,强调意识形态、社会历史、文化规范等因素对翻译活动的影响。通过考查中医药翻译文本的内部因素与超文本因素之间相互制约与影响的关系,可以深入了解中医药翻译文本英译中存在翻译问题的原因,从而为制定有效的多元化翻译策略与方法提供理论依据。

三、德国功能学派目的论与应用

1. 德国功能学派目的论

"目的论"的原文为"Skopos Theory",其中的"Skopos"为希腊语,意为"动机、目的、功能"。在莱斯文本类型理论基础上,20世纪70年代,师从莱斯的德国学者费米尔提出了翻译目的论,其核心概念是:决定翻译过程的最主要因素是整体翻译行为的目的。目的论将翻译行为的目的概括为三种：译者的基本目的、目的语环境中译文的交际目的和使用特定翻译策略或翻译程序的目的。在一般情况下，译文的交际目的比另外两个目的更为重要（Vermeer，1989：100）。译者在整个翻译过程中的参照系不应是"对等"翻译理论所注重的原文及其功能，而应是译文在译语文化环境中预期达到的一种或几种交际功能。因此，弄清楚翻译原文的目的以及译文的功能对于译者而言至关重要。在译者选择一定的文本信息来实现一定目的的过程中，译者为实现翻译目的，可以根据具体情境，选择增译、省译、重写等不同的翻译策略。

1991年，同样师从莱斯的另一名德国学者诺德提出了"功能+忠实"（function plus loyalty）的概念，大大丰富了"目的论"理论。她指出，"目的论"作为一个基本的翻译理论，当它被应用到具体翻译实践中去时，不能离开"忠诚"。所谓"忠诚"，应该包括尊重翻译过程发起者、原文作者、源语文化和译文读者。可见，"忠诚"原则一方面限制了译文功能的随意扩张，另一方面又增加了译者与有关各方对翻译任务的必要协商。诺德明确提出，译者应在分析原文的基础上，为实现译文预期功能进行必要的调整，包括删减甚至改写，使译文被译语系统所接受，达到与语篇类型和功能相一致的得体性，从而为决定处于特定语境的原文中哪些成分可以保留、哪些可以或必须根据译语语境进行调整甚至改写提供了标准（方梦之、毛忠明，2018：30）。

2. 中医药外宣翻译策略

中医药外宣翻译具有明确的翻译目的，即提升译文的海外接受度和传播效果，推动中医药文化海外传播，因此，"目的论"为制定中医药外宣翻译策略提供了理论基础。本教材采用广义的外宣翻译资料概念，即和中医药相关的所有应用文本。应用文本面向现实世界，以传达信息和施加影响为主，具有现实的预期要达到的目的或功能。这就要求译者以"内容"（信息型文本）或"效果"（感染型文本）为重，确定原语篇的语言特征是否能达到译文预期功能，如有相悖之处，应考虑基于译文读者的接受期望和译文的预期目的，采取得体的表达形式进行灵活翻译，对原文信息进行适当取舍，甚至改变原文的文本形式和风格，使译文语言对译语接收者产生有效的影响力。

第三节 中医药外宣翻译教学模式

为产出实现预期功能、符合行业规范、能被读者所接受的译文，构建以促进学生文本灵活变通翻译能力培养为导向的中医药翻译教学模式就显得尤为重要。本教程的文本教学设计理念以德国功能学派翻译理论为先导,以平行文本语料库为依托,以翻译策略为主干,以翻译任务为教学手段。

一、基于德国功能学派翻译理论实施"自上而下"的翻译教学

德国功能主义翻译理论代表人物诺德从文本功能的视角具体指明了翻译的主导方向,提倡采取"自上而下"的文本分析思维路径,即从文本较高层级到较低层级单位,对原文进行适应性变通,生产出"功能+忠诚"的译文(Nord,2005:43-143)。在解决好语用、文化层面的问题之后,大部分语言层面的问题将会迎刃而解(曹志建,2016:87)。中医药外宣翻译教学以德国功能学派翻译理论为依据,引导学生按照从语篇到段落,再到句子和词语的顺序,"自上而下"地对平行文本进行对比分析和翻译调整,实现译文的预期功能和目的。

1. 语篇层面

语篇层面的平行文本对比分析和翻译调整是中医药外宣翻译教学的首要环节。学生对比、分析源文本和平行文本在语篇特征上的差异,分析产生差异的社会文化背景、文本功能、目标受众、翻译目的等超文本因素原因,进而借鉴平行文本的语篇模式及体现样式,进行宏观语篇翻译调整。

所谓语篇(discourse 或 text)是指表达特定的交际功能的信息载体,以语篇为单位的翻译不仅追求译文与原文整体意义上的等值,注重对篇章结构和语用意义的分析,也关注篇章的语篇类型、翻译目的、译文的功能、译文读者等其他制约因素对翻译的影响(王国风:2014:129)。特定的语篇体裁(genre)通过纲要式结构(schematic structure)和体现样式(realizational patterns)两种方式体现。纲要式结构是指整个语篇有阶段、有步骤的结构,即篇章的整体框架,而体现样式则通常由特定的语言结构即模式化的句子来实现,体现术语专业程度、语言正式度以及作者和读者之间的心理距离。不同语篇体裁的排版、插图、字体等非语言因素也应考虑在内。汉英两种语言中,有些语篇体裁交际功能相同,但纲要式结构有所差异,而有些篇章的纲要式结构基本一致,但体现样式却不同,因此在翻译过程中需要进行相应调整。以汉英医药行业网上宣传资料为例,尽管汉英网上简介都具有信息功能,但纲要式结构有所不同,体现样式也有明显差异。如汉语简介通常采取第三人称,篇幅较长,小标题不多见,表格、图表更少见,长句和大词运用较多,文体正式度较高;而英语简介通常运用第一人称,从消费者视角选取实质性内容,借助小标题分清结构层次,每个部分重点突出,

善于运用图片、图表、视频等手段,词语多使用日常词汇,句子较为简短。

2. 段落、句子层面

完成语篇层面框架和语言结构调整后,须站在语篇的高度审视原文,围绕语篇的中心话题重构译文语篇脉络,继而构建各个分话题之间的并列、对比、转折、递进等逻辑关系,每一个一级分话题又可能由若干个二级分话题构成,以此类推(王树槐,2013:73–74)。段落是具有明确的始末标记、语义相对完整、交际功能相对独立的语篇单位,其基本特征是衔接与连贯。连贯是一种内在形式,是无形的,指语篇各个部分的语义连接应当通顺而流畅,而衔接是一种外在形式,是有形的,指语篇中语言成分之间的语义联系。可以说,连贯的语篇一定是衔接良好的,而表面衔接良好的语篇却未必连贯。篇章连贯性并不单纯依赖语言表面形式之间的联系而存在,而是取决于篇章的意义、概念和命题之间在逻辑上的联系程度。

英语重形合,注重形式逻辑,强调运用各种有形的连接手段达到语言形式上的连贯;而汉语重意合,注重以神统领,各个短句按时间或逻辑顺序逐步展开,体现的是内在逻辑上的连贯。此外,汉语和英语在主位推进模式上也有所不同,虽然它们的主语线性顺序大体相同,但在句法和语义上却存在重大区别(李运兴,2001:206)。通过借鉴英文平行文本的英文构句的关键词语和句式,有助于翻译时转变汉语思维,使译文尽量贴近英语作为母语人士的思维方式和谋篇构句的思路,从而译出逻辑清楚、通顺地道的英文。在对翻译中不明的逻辑关系进行调整的过程中,译者需要仔细分析汉语各个语义部分之间的内在逻辑,用合适的英语衔接手段表现出来,还需要根据实际情况重构主位推进模式,使译文合乎英语的表达习惯——逻辑清楚、语义完整、表达流畅。

3. 词语层面

翻译教学的最后环节是从词语层面进行对比分析和翻译调整。语篇逻辑和连贯除了与语篇自身的信息安排有关以外,还和译文读者的接受度相关,译文必须考虑到读者的接受习惯和对有关背景知识的了解程度,调整语句表达和词语的翻译,以贴近原文的表达意图和译文读者的接受语境(李运兴,2001:201)。汉英两种语言形式上区别很大,翻译总是存在着形和义的矛盾。词语翻译也是如此,译者必须尽最大努力再现原文的义,于是就在形和义之间纠结和选择。中医药术语是中医药翻译的重点和难点,翻译过程中,译者是采取注重形式的音译或直译,还是采用意译和释译等方法追求最大化传递原文信息,取决于诗学规范、文本功能、翻译目的、译者主体等多种因素。

二、基于文本分析提取与归纳多元化翻译策略

翻译策略是宏观理论连接翻译实践的必由之路,贯穿于整个翻译过程。本节讨论的翻译策略指的是文本策略。文本策略指语言层面的解决方案,多由译者来做出决定,包括常规解决方案和针对某些问题的宏观和微观上的解决方案。

1. 宏观翻译策略

中医药外宣翻译教学首先引导学生以语篇为翻译单位,通过平行文本对比分析,提取、归纳宏观翻译策略。宏观策略涉及整个文本,制约整个翻译过程,归化、异化、语义翻译、交际翻译、动态对等等概念皆属于此类。归化和异化翻译近年来是中医药翻译研究讨论的焦点。中西方对"异化"策略有着不同的理解,最初韦努蒂所说的"异化"策略是出于翻译伦理考虑的"文化策略",用来抵制欧美文化中心主义的流畅翻译规范。而"异化"一词在中国被缩小为"文本策略",连同"归化"策略,指译者针对两种文化和语言的差异,面对翻译目的、文本类型、作者意图、译入语读者等方面的不同而采取的两种不同的翻译策略。归化追求译文符合译入语文化和语言规范,是译文读者取向;异化追求保留原文文化和语言特色,是原文作者取向(都立澜、朱建平、洪梅,2020:2839)。

就中医药外宣翻译而言,因其文本类型主要是信息型或感染型,译者应以"内容"(信息型文本)或"效果"(感染型文本)为出发点,确定原语篇的语言特征是否为达到译文预期功能的得体手段,如有相悖之处,需在篇章结构、内容和语言形式上进行调整,运用节译、改译、编译等翻译策略,使译文对目标受众产生良好的影响力,取得最佳的传播效果。如汉英简介在体裁、内容和正式度上有明显差异,译者在翻译中医药企事业单位网上宣传资料的过程中,须遵循目的语文本规范,剔除与读者和目的不相关的信息,并将同类信息归在一起,运用西方读者习惯的表达,准确传递原文信息,并感染目标受众,使其采取行动。

2. 微观翻译策略

微观策略决定译文局部的具体的翻译方法,如增译、减译、词性转换法、加注等策略。中医药名词术语和四字词语是翻译的重点和难点,译者需根据译文预期功能,灵活运用直译、音译等异化策略,以及意译、释译等归化翻译策略。直译是指在不违背英语文化传统的前提下,在英译文中完全保留汉英词语的指称意义,以求译语在内容和形式上与原语相符的方法,如中医关于人体器官的许多名词术语的翻译基本上直接采用西医词汇(郑玲,2013:27)。音译法是指在英语译文中保留汉语的发音,以便

突出原文主要语言功能的翻译方法,对于为中国文化所专有、内涵独特、无法在英语中找到对应词语的中医药术语,通常采用音译,如"阴"和"阳"音译为"yin""yang"。为使译文与原文取得内容与形式的统一,同时又能帮助读者正确理解译文,翻译中医药术语时常采取直译或音译加释译的方法。意译是在无法或不宜保留原文形式的时候采取的趋向于达意的选择,在中医英语翻译中占有举足轻重的地位。中医药术语的翻译常常只译出其基本含义,而不拘泥于其具体的表达方式或修辞手法。译文译其意而舍其形,这既考虑到读者的感受,也为了顺应英语的行文习惯和规范。当然,中医药名词术语和四字词语的翻译方法的选择还要受到社会文化背景、诗学规范、文本功能、翻译目的等外在因素的影响和制约。

三、依托平行文本语料库开展翻译任务教学

中医药外宣翻译教学以平行文本语料库作为主要教学工具与依托,不仅能够增强翻译教学的操作性,而且有助于将以教师"教"为主的传统翻译教学转变成以学习者为中心的自主的、研究式的学习(夏天,2015:21)。学生对平行文本语料库提供的典型、真实、丰富的译例进行观察、分析和思考,分析和归纳目标文本在语言、文体等方面的主要特点,并与源语文本的对应特点相比较,从而在译文中再现这些特点,产出地道的、功能对等的译文(李德超、王克非,2009:55),有助于培养学生灵活的翻译技能,提高学生在真实场景下的翻译实践能力(熊兵,2015:9)。在这种情况下,平行文本可以被看作一种"规范文本"(Nord,2007:17-26)。任务式教学法以具体任务组织教学,学生在完成任务的过程中,学习翻译理论,了解翻译过程,掌握翻译策略,塑造价值观,以互动、交流、合作的方式,完成教师设定的任务。中医药外宣翻译教学按照翻译任务前、中、后三个阶段,划分为平行文本对比分析、翻译任务设计和小组合作实施三个环节。

1. 抓住重点做好平行文本对比分析

在正式实施每项翻译任务前,教师引导学生通过批判性阅读,对语料库提供的典型、真实、丰富的中西方译例进行观察、分析和思考,以帮助学生归纳中西方文本规范差异,领悟社会文化语境、意识形态、文本功能、目标受众与翻译目的对翻译策略选择的制约与限制作用,从而使其掌握如何灵活运用翻译方法和策略,按照"自上而下"的路径进行翻译调整。例如,在中医药科研论文文本分析中,将国内作者用英文译写的中医药科研论文与西方医学科研论文对比,帮助学生了解中西学术论文在语篇结构与语言惯例方面的差异,进而使其掌握如何借鉴西方医学论文规约,运用恰当的语言

策略,确保英文写译的论文传递的信息能为国外受众理解与认可,从而增强中医药学术话语的国际影响力;中医药新闻文本分析将国内与国外媒体的中医药英文新闻报道进行对比,重点帮助学生了解国外媒体新闻如何通过叙事视角、结构与语言来构建现实,传递意识形态,从而掌握如何借鉴西方常用的新闻文体结构与话语方式译写中医英文新闻,提升中医文化形象,增强中医药话语的国际影响力;企事业单位网页简介文本分析将中西方医药行业的网站宣传资料文本进行特征对比,重点分析如何从纲要结构和体现样式方面进行译文调整,并进行段落逻辑重构,以达到传递信息、感染海外受众、促进中医药文化海外传播的交际效果。在课堂讨论之后,教师指导学生进行专项训练和翻译练习,帮助学生及时掌握、巩固多元化翻译策略知识与技能。

2. 强化策略导向进行翻译任务设计

翻译任务布置环节重点培养学生选用变通翻译策略的能力。为此,设计任务时要求学生不能全译、机械翻译、逐字翻译,他们必须基于行业规范,根据任务的翻译目的、目标读者、文本类型等因素,选用全译、节译、编译、改译等恰当的翻译策略,进行灵活翻译和译写。翻译任务包括但不限于以下内容:① 从中医药重点期刊中选择一篇适合在 SCI 期刊发表的中文科研论文、综述或临床报告,译成英文,或用英文完成一篇论文;② 选择《中华人民共和国中医药法》和《新型冠状病毒肺炎针灸干预的指导意见》某个段落进行翻译,要求体现公文英译规范,易于海外读者理解与接受;③ 从《中国日报》(*China Daily*) 或《人民日报》海外版(*People's Daily*) 选择一篇中医药英文新闻报道,以海外普通读者易于接受的话语方式进行编译;④ 从中文科普读物《奇妙中医药:家庭保健顾问》中选择海外读者可能感兴趣的一篇进行翻译,并进行适当的内容和形式调整;⑤ 翻译一篇中成药说明书,要求准确传递信息,产生预期交际效果,推动中医药文化的传播;⑥ 将一篇企事业单位网页中文介绍译成英文,为潜在海外用户提供准确信息,并产生吸引力与感染力。教师在布置每项任务时,会在翻译任务作业单上明确给出翻译目的和要求,让学生自己思考如何根据译文预期功能选用适当的翻译策略。

3. 译、评结合指导小组实施任务

任务教学以小组合作的形式组织实施。合作学习被誉为"近几十年来最重要的和最成功的教学改革",是指为促进学习者提高学习效果、共同完成学习任务的一种学习方式(Vermette, 1994: 255 - 260)。学生在合作学习法的指导下,以小组活动和同伴活动的形式在翻译过程中进行交际,共享信息、相互帮助,合作评估自己的努力和进步(王笃勤,2002: 138 - 140)。"译"和"评"是翻译教学的两条线(徐姚伟、周领顺,2020:2),教师围绕以上两个方面,要求学生合作完成上述翻译任务,每项任务根据其复杂程度,给予1~2周的时间完成。首先是构建小组专题语料库,小组每位成员根据翻译任务要求搜集平行文本,构建小组专项平行文本语料库,小组进行讨论互相启发,提取与归纳目的语文本的体裁结构、语篇模式和语篇脉络,归纳文本规范,每位成员借鉴文本规范完成翻译初稿。其次是译文评价的过程,由自评、互评和教师评价三部分构成。自评过程中,每位学生对照教师给出的翻译评价标准和错误分析表进行自我评级和错误分析;小组成员开展同伴互评,并互相给出评级和具体评价意见,学生根据自评和互评结果修改自己的初稿,完成个人自我评估报告;教师对每位学生的修改稿进行批改并给予评级,对自我评估报告进行反馈。最后是小组陈述环节,每个小组汇报本组的翻译任务实施情况,特别对小组专项语料库建构过程和变通翻译策略选用的合理性进行说明,教师最后总结点评。

第四节　翻译练习与任务

一、翻译练习

以下是《灵枢·九针十二原》一段的三个译文,比较各译文的风格和翻译策略,并结合中医药外宣翻译的四个特征对其译文的合理性和传播效果进行分析。①

今夫五脏之有疾也,譬犹刺也,犹污也,犹结也,犹闭也。刺虽久,犹可拔也;污虽久,犹可雪也;结虽久,犹可解也;闭虽久,犹可决也。或言久疾之不可取者,非其说也。

译文1:The occurrence of visceral disease is quite similar to the state of a human body that has been thorned, an object that has been contaminated, a piece of rope that has been knotted or a river that has been blocked. A deeply lodged thorn can be pulled out, a long contaminated object can be cleaned, a long knitted knot can be undone and a long blocked river can be dredged. Some people regard stubborn diseases as incurable, this view is incorrect.

译文2:The occurrence of visceral disease is just like the state of a thorned human

---

① 译文选自:李照国.中医英语翻译技巧[M].北京:人民卫生出版社,1997:266-268.

body, a contaminated object, a piece of knotted rope or a blocked river which, though long troubled, can still be overcome. Thus, it is incorrect to regard stubborn disease as incurable.

译文 3：The occurrence of visceral disease is just like the appearance of any problem which, though difficult, can be solved later on. Thus, stubborn diseases are also curable.

二、翻译任务

以小组为单位，讨论在翻译学习或翻译实践中接触的中医药翻译文本类型、你所采取的翻译策略与实现的传播效果，并思考如何讲好中医药文化故事，塑造具有亲切感、感召力的国家形象。

三、拓展阅读

[1] 高芸. 中医外宣翻译理论与教学实践［M］. 上海：上海交通大学出版社，2023.

[2] 李长栓. 非文学翻译理论与实践［M］. 北京：中国对外翻译出版公司，2004.

[3] 张健. 外宣翻译导论［M］. 北京：国防工业出版社，2013.

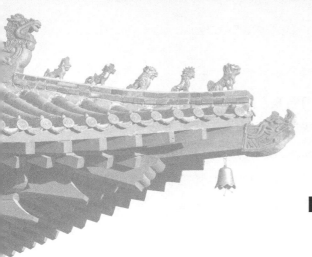

第二章
中医药政府文书英译

  政府公文是行政机关在行政管理过程中所形成的具有法定效力和规范体式的公务文书,有多种不同类型,如指示、决议、公告、通知、报告等。译成外文的政府公文通常是涉及国际社会共同关心的领域,体现政府立场或者介绍我国政府重大举措的较为正式的文本,如白皮书、政府工作报告等(胡洁,2010:62)。其中,白皮书是国际公认的官方文件,用于介绍一国政府在重大事件和问题上的原则立场、政策主张和进展,也是政府文献中传达国家和政府原则立场最具代表性的一类文件(赵家明,2022:22)。因此,白皮书英译既要准确传递源语中的文本信息,增进国际社会对中国的了解,又要表达中国政府的立场和观点(杨冬青,2013:112),向国际社会展现积极正面的国家形象。白皮书等政府公文在语言特征上,行文庄重、用词严谨、逻辑缜密,与普通文体和非正式文体存在明显差异,因此在翻译时也需要注意其文体特点,选择能体现源语特点的篇章结构、句式和词汇,充分体现出其严肃、庄重、正式的文体特点。

第一节 语料导入

  本节中文语料选择了国务院新闻办公室 2016 年发布的《中国的中医药》白皮书①

---

  ① 来源:http://www.scio.gov.cn/zfbps/zfbps_2279/202207/t20220704_130520.html,搜索日期:2022-09-01。

和 2020 年发布的《抗击新冠肺炎疫情的中国行动》白皮书①（以下简称《抗击新冠》），英文语料则为 2013 年世界卫生组织（WHO）发布的《世界卫生组织传统医学战略 2014—2023》（*WHO Traditional Medicine Strategy: 2014 - 2023*②，以下简称《传统医学战略》），以及 2022 年美国国会发布的《大麻作为管控物质的演变以及联邦与州之间的政策差距》白皮书（*The Evolution of Marijuana as a Controlled Substance and the Federal-State Policy Gap*③，以下简称《大麻法案》）。《传统医学战略》虽不是常规意义上的白皮书，但它是由世界卫生组织这样的国际机构发布的权威报告，在格式和语言上均具有较高的规范性。本节仅列出用于语篇分析的《中国的中医药》和《大麻法案》部分内容，段落和词语分析语料在第三节、第四节分别呈现，本节不再列出。

一、中文语料

中医药历史发展脉络④

在远古时代，中华民族的祖先发现了一些动植物可以解除病痛，积累了一些用药知识。随着人类的进化，开始有目的地寻找防治疾病的药物和方法，所谓"神农尝百草""药食同源"，就是当时的真实写照。夏代（约前 2070—前 1600）酒和商代（前 1600—前 1046）汤液的发明，为提高用药效果提供了帮助。进入西周时期（前 1046—前 771），开始有了食医、疾医、疡医、兽医的分工。春秋战国（前 770—前 221）时期，扁鹊总结前人经验，提出"望、闻、问、切"四诊合参的方法，奠定了中医临床诊断和治疗的基础。秦汉时期（前 221—公元 220）的中医典籍《黄帝内经》，系统论述了人的生理、病理、疾病以及"治未病"和疾病治疗的原则及方法，确立了中医学的思维模式，标志着从单纯的临床经验积累发展到了系统理论总结阶段，形成了中医药理论体系框架。东汉时期，张仲景的《伤寒杂病论》，提出了外感热病（包括瘟疫等传染病）的诊治原则和方法，论述了内伤杂病的病因、病证、诊法、治疗、预防等辨证规律和原则，确立了辨证论治的理论和方法体系。同时期的《神农本草经》，概括论述了君臣佐使、七

---

① 来源：http://www.scio.gov.cn/zfbps/ndhf/2020n/202207/t20220704_130649.html，搜索日期：2022 - 09 - 1。
② 来源：https://iris.who.int/bitstream/handle/10665/92455/9789245506096_chi.pdf，搜索日期：2022 - 12 - 17。
③ 来源：https://crsreports.congress.gov/product/pdf/R/R44782，搜索日期：2022 - 12 - 18。
④ 选自《中国的中医药》白皮书第一部分"中医药的历史发展"中的第一小节。

情合和、四气五味等药物配伍和药性理论,对于合理处方、安全用药、提高疗效具有十分重要的指导作用,为中药学理论体系的形成与发展奠定了基础。东汉末年,华佗创制了麻醉剂"麻沸散",开创了麻醉药用于外科手术的先河。西晋时期(265—317),皇甫谧的《针灸甲乙经》,系统论述了有关脏腑、经络等理论,初步形成了经络、针灸理论。唐代(618—907),孙思邈提出的"大医精诚",体现了中医对医道精微、心怀至诚、言行诚谨的追求,是中华民族高尚的道德情操和卓越的文明智慧在中医药中的集中体现,是中医药文化的核心价值理念。明代(1368—1644),李时珍的《本草纲目》在世界上首次对药用植物进行了科学分类,创新发展了中药学的理论和实践,是一部药物学和博物学巨著。清代(1644—1911),叶天士的《温热论》提出了温病和时疫的防治原则及方法,形成了中医药防治瘟疫(传染病)的理论和实践体系。清代中期以来,特别是民国时期,随着西方医学的传入,一些学者开始探索中西医药学汇通、融合。

二、英文语料

Historical Background of Federal Marijuana Policy[①]
(联邦大麻政策的历史背景)

To understand the evolution of U. S. marijuana control and the current marijuana policy gap between the states and the federal government, it is important to examine the history of marijuana as a controlled substance in the United States.

Early 20th Century

Prior to 1937, growing and using marijuana was legal under federal law. During the course of promoting federal legislation to control marijuana, Henry Anslinger, the first commissioner of the Federal Bureau of Narcotics (FBN), and others submitted testimony to Congress regarding the immorality and harms of marijuana use, claiming that it incited violent and insane behavior. Among other observations, Commissioner Anslinger noted that "the major criminal in the United States is the drug addict; that of all the offenses committed against the laws of this country, the narcotic addict is the most frequent offender." States had already begun to ban the possession of marijuana during this time. The federal government created a de facto ban of marijuana under the Marihuana Tax Act of 1937 (MTA; P. L. 75 - 238). The MTA imposed a high-cost transfer tax stamp on

---

① 选自《大麻法案》第一部分。

marijuana sales, but these stamps were rarely issued by the federal government.

Early 20th Century Marijuana Control

In the early 20th century, enforcement of drug laws was primarily the responsibility of local police, and the Federal Bureau of Narcotics (FBN) occasionally assisted. Due to reduced appropriations during the Great Depression, the FBN budget and the number of narcotic agents declined and remained low for years. Publicity and warnings of the dangers of narcotics, in particular marijuana, were primary methods of drug control for the FBN. In seeking federal control of marijuana and uniform narcotic laws, Commissioner Anslinger and public officials from some states made personal appeals to civic groups and legislators and pushed for, and received, editorial support in newspapers; some newspapers maintained a steady stream of anti-marijuana messaging in the 1930s.

Mid-20th Century

In the decades that followed the enactment of the MTA, Congress continued to pass drug control legislation and further criminalized drug use. For example, the Boggs Act (P. L. 82 − 255), passed in 1951, established mandatory prison sentences for some drug offenses, while the Narcotic Control Act (P. L. 84 − 728) in 1956 further increased penalties for drug offenses, including marijuana offenses. In conjunction with growing support for a medical approach to addressing drug abuse, there was a strong emphasis on law enforcement control of drugs, including marijuana—which was gaining popularity as a recreational drug. Congress shifted the constitutional basis for drug control from its taxing authority to its power to regulate interstate commerce, and in 1968 the FBN merged with the Bureau of Drug Abuse Control and was transferred from Treasury to the Department of Justice (DOJ). Three years later, President Richard Nixon would declare a war on drugs.

Congress and President Nixon enhanced federal control of drugs through the enactment of comprehensive federal drug laws—including the CSA, enacted as Title II of the Comprehensive Drug Abuse Prevention and Control Act of 1970 (P. L. 91 − 513). The CSA placed the control of marijuana and other plant and chemical substances under federal jurisdiction regardless of state regulations and laws. In designating marijuana as a Schedule I controlled substance, this legislation officially prohibited the manufacture, distribution, dispensation, and possession of marijuana except for purposes of sanctioned research.

. . .

Marijuana, Late 20th Century and Beyond

While heroin and cocaine were the primary drugs of concern for federal law enforcement during the 1970s and 80s (respectively), marijuana was also a target of the substantial investment in enforcement during the federal government's "war on drugs". In the 1980s, marijuana arrests were a large part of federal drug enforcement, and there are some federal crime data available to illustrate this. The percentage of federal drug offenders charged with marijuana violations was 24% in 1980, increased to 40% in 1982, and decreased to 26% in 1986. Among federal drug offenders (12,285) charged with marijuana violations (3,221) in 1986, 70% were charged with distribution, manufacture, or importation, while the remaining 30% were charged with simple possession. Today, the percentage of federal drug offenders charged with marijuana violations is much lower—in FY 2020, 7% of federal drug offenders were marijuana offenders.

第二节　篇章的翻译

政府文书往往遵循统一规范的格式,结构严谨,不同的公文类型有不同的格式要求,本节聚焦以白皮书为代表的政府公文的篇章翻译。

一、篇章的对比分析

1. 纲要式结构

1）整体篇章结构

在宏观结构上,白皮书采用正式报告的行文格式,如标题+正文+结语(+附录),也包括发文机构、发布时间等公文要素。白皮书的正文部分根据其目的和内容不同,篇章结构不尽相同,大多包含引言、相关问题的社会背景,如对某一问题的历史回顾,或对其现状的分析,也往往包括针对这一问题所采取的措施或对策,以及对未来的展望或建议等。

《中国的中医药》是中国政府根据 WHO《传统医学战略》提出的战略目标,结合中国国情,将中医药发展上升为国家战略,研究制定的中国中医药发展战略。该白皮书系统介绍了中医药的发展脉络及其特点,阐述了中国发展中医药的国家政策和主要措施,展示了中医药的科学价值和文化特点,其正文结构如表 2-1 所示。

表 2-1 《中国的中医药》正文结构

目　　录	内　　容
前言	引言
一、中医药的历史发展	历史回顾
二、中国发展中医药的政策措施	措施
三、中医药的传承与发展	
四、中医药国际交流与合作	展望和建议
结束语	结语

《抗击新冠》白皮书是在 2020 年初,新冠疫情成为全球公共卫生紧急事件,在全球引发大面积流行的背景下发布的。中国政府果断采取严格的防控措施,有效阻断了新冠疫情在中国的蔓延,疫情防控阻击战取得了重大战略成果。中国国务院新闻办公室发布《抗击新冠》白皮书,是为了记录中国抗击疫情的艰辛历程,分享中国疫情防控和医疗救治的有效做法,介绍中国人民历经疫情磨难的感受和体会,传递团结合作、战胜疫情的信心和力量,其正文结构如表 2-2 所示。

表 2-2 《抗击新冠》正文结构

目　　录	内　　容
前言	引言
一、中国抗击疫情的艰辛历程	历史回顾
二、防控和救治两个战场协同作战	措施
三、凝聚抗击疫情的强大力量	心得体会
四、共同构建人类卫生健康共同体	展望和建议

《传统医学战略》根据世界卫生大会关于传统医学的决议制定,于2014年5月24日在世界卫生组织第67届世界卫生大会上审议并通过,旨在支持会员国通过掌握、利用传统医学,推动卫生保健事业发展,提升人民健康和福祉;研究、监管传统医学产品、技术服务的提供者和实践,酌情将产品和服务纳入卫生系统,促进传统和补充医学的安全、有效使用。《传统医学战略》为每项目标规定了若干行动指南,以具体指导会员国、合作伙伴、利益方以及世界卫生组织,并支持会员国根据本国的发展能力和重点以及相关法规制定和实施战略计划,其正文结构如表2-3所示。

表2-3 《传统医学战略》正文结构

目　　　录	内　　　容
1. Introduction	引言
2. Global progress	已有成就
3. Global review of T&CM	现状分析
4. Strategic objectives, strategic directions and strategic actions	措施
5. Implementing the strategy	实施和意义

《大麻法案》白皮书是美国国会研究服务部在2022年4月发布的。《大麻法案》在美国众议院通过大麻在全美合法化法案的背景下出台,全面回顾了美国有关大麻管制的联邦立法情况和州立法情况,分析了联邦政府和各州政府在对待大麻问题上的政策存在的差异,并指出在过去的25年中联邦政府和州政府在大麻立法上的差异增大,这一政策上的不同对个人和商业活动造成的困扰,并提出将大麻从联邦《受控物质法》中删除的建议,其正文结构如表2-4所示。

表2-4 《大麻法案》正文结构

目　　　录	内　　　容
1. Introduction	引言
2. Historical background of federal Marijuana policy	历史回顾
3. The federal status of Marijuana and the expanding policy gap with states	现状分析
4. Federal response to state divergence	

续　表

目　　录	内　　容
5. Select outcomes of state Marijuana legalization	产生的后果
6. Employment and educational consequences of the Marijuana policy gap for individuals	
7. International policy context and response	国际形势
8. Select issues for Congress——The path forward	展望和建议
9. Conclusion	结语

2）历史回顾部分篇章结构

因篇幅限制,此处仅选择《中国的中医药》与《大麻法案》两份文件中的历史回顾部分进行对比分析。历史回顾是白皮书中较为常见的一个组成部分,通过对相关问题的历史发展过程进行简要介绍,为读者提供相关问题的背景知识。

汉英语料都按照时间顺序进行历史回顾,但采用的结构不尽相同。中文语料只有一个相对较长的段落,按照从远古到近代的时间顺序,以并列式结构,用精练的语言高度概括了不同朝代的历史时期中医药的发展,完整呈现了中医药形成—发展—完善的过程(见表2-5)。英文语料首句是总起句,然后以三个时间段为小标题,分为8个段落进行论述。每个段落通常采用总分结构,每一段的主要内容通常以主题句(topic sentence)的形式出现在段首,再以支撑句/扩展句(supporting sentence)对主题句进行论证和补充说明,为主题句提供事实、事例、数据等论据。

2. 体现样式

本部分同样以《中国的中医药》和《大麻法案》两份白皮书作为语料,分析两者在历史回顾部分体现样式上的区别。

1）时间展开方式

汉英语料虽然都对所讨论主题的历史发展进行回顾和梳理,但在具体时间阶段的划分上,所采用的标准不尽相同。在中文语料《中国的中医药》中,中医药的发展历程历时三千多年,时间跨度很大,采用的是传统的中国历史的记录方法,以朝代更替为自然的历史节点,按照不同的历史朝代进行梳理,遵循从远古到夏商周,再到秦汉、两晋、唐、明清,直至近代的顺序,叙述了中医药产生、发展、完善的整个过程(见表2-5)。

表 2-5 中医药历史发展脉络

时 期	主 要 成 就
远古时期	积累初步的用药知识
夏商	酒和汤液的发明提高了药效
西周	食医、疾医、疡医、兽医的分工
春秋战国	扁鹊提出四诊合参的方法,奠定临床诊断和治疗的基础
秦汉	《黄帝内经》的出现,形成中医药理论体系框架
东汉	张仲景《伤寒杂病论》,确立辨证论治的理论和方法 《神农本草经》,奠定中药学理论体系的形成和发展 华佗,开创麻沸散用于外科手术的先河
西晋	皇甫谧《针灸甲乙经》,初步形成经络、针灸理论
唐代	孙思邈"大医精诚",形成中医药文化的核心价值理念
明代	李时珍《本草纲目》,对药用植物进行分类,创新发展了中药学
清代	叶天士《温热论》,形成中医药防治瘟疫的理论和实践
清中期至今	中西医药学的汇通、融合

美国对大麻管控政策的历史发展过程相对较短,主要集中在 20 世纪,在进行历史回顾时,则是以重要法案的出台为主要标志,如第一阶段为 20 世纪早期,便是以 1937 年《大麻税法》(Marihuana Tax Act)的出台为重要标志,在此之前大麻在联邦法律中处于合法地位,而该法案开始对大麻进行了实际上的禁止;在此之后的第二阶段即 20 世纪中期,一系列重要法案被发布,如 1951 年的《博格斯法》(Boggs Act)以及 1970 年的《受控物质法》(Controlled Substances Act)等,加强了联邦立法层面对大麻的控制;再到第三阶段,20 世纪后期,大麻成为联邦政府"毒品之战"的打击目标(见表 2-6)。

表 2-6 美国大麻管控立法

时 期	管 控 状 态
Early 20th century	Legal under federal law
Mid-20th century	Continued to pass control legislation and criminalized drug use A: Controlled Substances Act B: The Shafer Commission
Late 20th century and beyond	A target of federal government's "war on drugs"

2）内容的呈现方式

中文语料从宏观的视角,对每个历史阶段中医药发展的主要成就进行高度精炼的概括,而英文语料采用事实、事例、引言、数据等多种方法进行阐述,如语料的第二段中"Among other observations, Commissioner Anslinger noted that 'the major criminal in the United States is the drug addict...'",直接引用了联邦麻醉品管理委员会委员安斯林格对药物成瘾问题的看法;又如以具体数据说明20世纪末联邦政府对打击大麻犯罪的力度。

3）脚注的使用

此外,我们还注意到英语语料中频繁地使用脚注,对正文中涉及的内容进行补充,说明细节或者说明出处。使用脚注既可以保证正文部分行文流畅,又可以为正文中的相关内容补充必要的细节或解释说明,便于读者理解,也可以对正文中提及的内容表明出处,使论述显得更加真实可靠。下面以中英文语料中的开头部分为例进行对比说明。

[例1] 在远古时代,中华民族的祖先发现了一些动植物可以解除病痛,积累了一些用药知识。随着人类的进化,开始有目的地寻找防治疾病的药物和方法,所谓"神农尝百草""药食同源",就是当时的真实写照。

对比句:Prior to 1937, growing and using marijuana was legal under federal law.[9] During the course of promoting federal legislation to control marijuana, Henry Anslinger, the first commissioner of the Federal Bureau of Narcotics (FBN)[10], and others submitted testimony to Congress regarding the immorality and harms of marijuana use, claiming that it incited violent and insane behavior[11].

---

9 States regulated marijuana, and some banned it prior to 1937.

10 In 1930, the Federal Bureau of Narcotics (FBN) was established within the U. S. Treasury Department to handle narcotics enforcement.

11 See statements by H. J. Anslinger, Commissioner of Narcotics, Federal Bureau of Narcotics, U. S. Department of the Treasury, and Dr. James C. Munch, before the U. S. Congress, House Committee on Ways and Means, *Taxation of Marihuana,* 75th Cong., 1st sess., April 27 – 30, May 4, 1937 HRG – 1837 – WAM – 0002.

分析:英文语料中多次使用脚注,对其中出现的相关知识进行补充或者提供出处,如脚注9补充说明有些州在1937年前已经开始禁止大麻,脚注10对FBN这一机构的建立提供了更具体的信息,脚注11对所提及的史实提供了详细出处,使读者可以更进一步了解文中的相关背景知识,也使得论述更加真实可靠。对于中文语料中

"神农尝百草""药食同源"这样的表述,翻译中如果也能以脚注的形式提供更多的信息,则会更便于不熟悉中国和中医文化的国外读者更好地理解其内涵。

二、篇章翻译的特点与策略

白皮书由政府或权威机构发布,具有高于读者的权威性和明确性,因此译文在篇章结构上也应尽量向原文靠近,不可任意添加或删减原文内容(胡洁,2010：72)。我们注意到,《中国的中医药》和《抗击新冠》的译者在英译过程中,根据英文段落主题集中、篇幅短小的特点,在译文段落的分配上进行适当的调整,以符合英文读者的阅读习惯,提高他们对白皮书的接受程度。例2和例3分别是《中国的中医药》和《抗击新冠》的部分英文译文。

[例2]　在远古时代,中华民族的祖先发现了一些动植物可以解除病痛,积累了一些用药知识。随着人类的进化,开始有目的地寻找防治疾病的药物和方法,所谓"神农尝百草""药食同源",就是当时的真实写照。夏代(约前2070—前1600)酒和商代(前1600—前1046)汤液的发明,为提高用药效果提供了帮助。进入西周时期(前1046—前771),开始有了食医、疾医、疡医、兽医的分工。春秋战国(前770—前221)时期,扁鹊总结前人经验,提出"望、闻、问、切"四诊合参的方法,奠定了中医临床诊断和治疗的基础。

译文：In remote antiquity, the ancestors of the Chinese nation chanced to find that some creatures and plants could serve as remedies for certain ailments and pains, and came to gradually master their application. As time went by, people began to actively seek out such remedies and methods for preventing and treating diseases. Sayings like "Shennong (Celestial Farmer) tasting a hundred herbs" and "food and medicine coming from the same source" are characteristic of those years.

The discovery of alcohol in the Xia Dynasty (c. 2070 – 1600 BC) and the invention of herbal decoction in the Shang Dynasty (1600 – 1046 BC) rendered medicines more effective.

In the Western Zhou Dynasty (1046 – 771 BC), doctors began to be classified into four categories—dietician, physician, doctor of decoctions and veterinarian.

During the Spring and Autumn and Warring States Period (770 – 221 BC), Bian Que drew on the experience of his predecessors and put forward the four diagnostic methods—inspection, auscultation & olfaction, inquiry, and palpation, laying the foundation for TCM diagnosis and treatment.

　　分析：译者在英译《中国的中医药》时，注意到了英语段落通常较为短小、主题集中的特点，如果将原有的一整段中文直接翻译为一个英语段落，无疑会显得过于冗长，因此在翻译时，基本按照表2-5中的朝代划分，将原文的一个自然段划分为11个段落，每个段落突出一个历史时期中医药的发展和成就，显得主题更加清晰，层次分明，也能使读者较快地对中医药发展的重要时期产生直观的认识。因篇幅限制，此处只展示了所选语料译文的1~4段。可以看出，译者按照从远古时期—夏商—西周—春秋战国的历史发展顺序，以每个历史时期为节点，单独划分为一个段落，在结构上更加清晰。

　　[例3] **及时总结推广行之有效的诊疗方案**。坚持边实践、边研究、边探索、边总结、边完善，在基于科学认知和证据积累的基础上，将行之有效的诊疗技术和科技研究成果纳入诊疗方案。先后制修订7版新冠肺炎诊疗方案，3版重型、危重型病例诊疗方案，2版轻型、普通型管理规范，2版康复者恢复期血浆治疗方案，1版新冠肺炎出院患者主要功能障碍康复治疗方案，提高了医疗救治工作的科学性和规范性。最新的第7版新冠肺炎诊疗方案增加病理改变内容，增补和调整临床表现、诊断标准、治疗方法和出院标准等，并纳入无症状感染者可能具有感染性、康复者恢复期血浆治疗等新发现。目前，第7版诊疗方案已被多个国家借鉴和采用。强化治愈出院患者隔离管理和健康监测，加强复诊复检和康复，实现治疗、康复和健康监测一体化全方位医疗服务。注重孕产妇、儿童等患者差异性诊疗策略，实现不同人群诊疗方案的全覆盖。①

　　译文：Reviewing diagnostic and therapeutic plans and applying effective ones on a broad scale. China's diagnostic and therapeutic plans for COVID-19 have been developed and improved through clinical practice, medical research, experimentation and regular reviews. Based on scientific knowledge and accumulated evidence, R&D results and the diagnostic and therapeutic regimens that proved effective were incorporated in the national diagnosis and treatment plans. These include seven versions of the diagnosis and treatment protocol, three editions of the protocol for severe and critical cases, two editions of the manual for mild case management, two editions of convalescent plasma

---

　　① 选自《抗击新冠》白皮书第二部分"防控和救治两个战场协同作战"第三小节"全力救治患者、拯救生命"第四段。

therapy treatment protocol, and one rehabilitation treatment program for patients discharged from hospitals. All these protocols and plans have contributed to science-based treatment of patients and the establishment of standards for medical treatment.

In Diagnosis and Treatment Protocol for COVID-19 (Trial Version 7), information on pathological changes, clinical symptoms, criteria for diagnosis, therapies, and criteria for patient discharge was added or updated. The protocol states that asymptomatic cases may be contagious. It also notes that plasma from convalescent cases may work in treating the infected. This edition has been adopted or used for reference in a number of countries.

Concerning discharged patients, quarantining, monitoring of their health and rehabilitation, and reexamination and re-testing have all been strengthened. Integrated medical services covering treatment, rehabilitation and health monitoring have been put in place. Differentiated treatment approaches have been adopted for children and pregnant women, among other groups.

分析：在中文原文中，以"及时总结推广行之有效的诊疗方案"作为该段的主题句，介绍了中国在诊疗方案方面的积极做法。论述实际上是分了三个层次进行的，首先介绍了中国总结并先后推出了 7 版诊疗方案的情况；其次着重介绍了第 7 版的诊疗方案；最后是对康复监测和诊疗方案全覆盖的介绍。在译文中，译者将原文的一个段落按照论述的三个层次划分为三个小段，使每一小段的主题更显集中，层次清晰，长度也更为适中。

第三节　段落的翻译

白皮书是一种非常正式的文体形式，在段落和句法层面常常表现为包含长而复杂的句式，这一点在中文和英文语料中均较为显著。但是，相比而言，英语是一种形合的语言，因此句子在语法结构上较为严谨，有明显的主谓结构，通过从句、独立结构等对主句进行修饰和补充，并使用关联词表明句子之间的逻辑关系。而汉语是一种意合的语言，一个句子往往包含多个以逗号连接的短句，结构上相对较为松散，有些句子甚至没有明显的主语。因此在翻译时，须采用不同的翻译方法对原句进行调整，以达到更好的翻译效果。

一、段落的对比分析

1. 主语省略句

汉语为主题显著语言,因此汉语中普遍存在无主语句,只要句意连贯通畅,并不会影响中文读者的理解,对句法结构的要求并不严格,表现出开放性和松散性。而英语为主语显著语言,要求句子遵循严格的句法结构,除少数特定句式外,均要求有确定的主谓结构,主语的变化往往引起谓语动词的相应变化。

[例1] 随着人类的进化,开始有目的地寻找防治疾病的药物和方法,所谓"神农尝百草""药食同源",就是当时的真实写照。[①]

对比句:Congress and President Nixon enhanced federal control of drugs through the enactment of comprehensive federal drug laws—including the CSA, enacted as Title II of the Comprehensive Drug Abuse Prevention and Control Act of 1970 (P. L. 91 – 513) ... In designating marijuana as a Schedule I controlled substance, this legislation officially prohibited the manufacture, distribution, dispensation, and possession of marijuana except for purposes of sanctioned research. [②]

分析:汉语中有一类泛指人称句,表示劝告、警告、行为指示或是对一种社会现象的描述和评论,往往可以省略主语(杨丰宁,2006:113)。中文句的前半句显然属于这种情况,省略了"人们"这一泛指人称。后半句则以"神农尝百草"和"药食同源"为主语。英语对比句中可以看出主谓关系清楚确定,第一句以"Congress and President Nixon"作为主语,而在第二句中用"this legislation"代指上文提到的CSA,保持了信息的连贯性。

[例2] 坚持中西医结合、中西药并用,发挥中医药治未病、辨证施治、多靶点干预的独特优势,全程参与深度介入疫情防控,从中医角度研究确定病因病基、治则治法,形成了覆盖医学观察期、轻型、普通型、重型、危重型、恢复期发病全过程的中医诊疗规范和技术方案,在全国范围内全面推广使用。[③]

---

① 选自《中国的中医药》白皮书第一部分"中医药的历史发展"第一小节"中医药历史发展脉络"第一段。
② 选自《大麻法案》第二部分"历史回顾"第二小节"二十世纪中期"第二段。
③ 选自《抗击新冠》白皮书第二部分"防控和救治两个战场协同作战"第三小节"全力救治患者、拯救生命"第五段。

对比句：① It is increasingly recognised that safe and effective T&CM could contribute to the health of our populations. ② One of the most significant questions raised about T&CM in recent years is how it might contribute to universal health coverage by improving service delivery in the health system, particularly PHC: patient accessibility to health services, and greater awareness of health promotion and disease prevention are key issues here. ③ Insurance coverage of T&CM products, practices and practitioners varies widely from full inclusion within insurance plans to total exclusion, with consumers having to pay for all T&CM out of pocket. ①

分析：汉语中多以话题为核心，而英语中则以主语为核心，有明显的主谓或主系表结构。在中文句中，核心话题是中医的作用，句中包含多个短句，且均没有明显的主语结构，而是由多个动宾结构组成，如"坚持……，发挥……，参与……，确定……，形成……，全面推广……"。而英语中则使用多种句式结构，如①句中使用了形式主语"It is .... that ..."，②③两句主语部分较长，分别是"one of the most significant questions raised about T&CM in recent years"，以及"insurance coverage of T&CM products, practices and practitioners"，但主语中心词均非常明确，分别是"questions"和"insurance coverage"，突出信息的重点。

2. 连动句

连动句是汉语中较为常见的一种句式形式，句子中往往存在两个以上的动词或动词词组作为谓语，且同属于一个主语，动词之间有先后、目的、因果、方式、条件等不同的语义关系。英语中则更强调句法形式和逻辑关系，句子中虽可能存在多个动词，但往往以一个动词作为谓语动词，而其他的动词则围绕谓语动词，以不定式结构、分词短语、介词短语等形式出现。

[例3] 秦汉时期（前221—公元220）的中医典籍《黄帝内经》系统论述了人的生理、病理、疾病以及"治未病"和疾病治疗的原则及方法，确立了中医学的思维模式，标志着从单纯的临床经验积累发展到了系统理论总结阶段，形成了中医药理论体系框架。②

对比句：In the decades that followed the enactment of the MTA, Congress continued to pass drug control legislation and further criminalized drug use. For example,

---

① 选自《传统医学战略》第四部分"战略目标、战略方向和战略行动"中的第三个战略目标第一段。

② 选自《中国的中医药》白皮书第一部分"中医药的历史发展"第一小节"中医药历史发展脉络"第一段。

the Boggs Act (P. L. 82 - 255), passed in 1951, established mandatory prison sentences for some drug offenses, while the Narcotic Control Act (P. L. 84 - 728) in 1956 further increased penalties for drug offenses, including marijuana offenses. ①

分析：中文句中,主语为"中医典籍《黄帝内经》",其后为四个连续的动词:"系统论述了""确立了""标志着""形成了",在句意上层层递进,先论述《黄帝内经》一书的主要内容和特点,再进一步论述其在中医发展史上的重要意义。而在英语对比句中,第一句为简单句,主谓结构明显,第二句以"for example"说明是对上句的举例说明的逻辑关系。这句前半句的谓语动词为"established",而动词前的"passed in 1951"则是作为过去分词短语,说明"the Boggs Act"通过的时间,后半句为"while"引导的并列从句,用主谓结构引入新的信息。可见,第二个句子中,多个动词分别充当不同的语法成分,语法结构严谨,层次清晰。

［例4］ 医疗救治始终以提高收治率和治愈率、降低感染率和病亡率的"两提高""两降低"为目标,坚持集中患者、集中专家、集中资源、集中救治"四集中"原则,坚持中西医结合,实施分类救治、分级管理。②

对比句： Mindful of the traditions and customs of peoples and communities, Member States should consider how T&CM, including self-health care, might support disease prevention or treatment, health maintenance and health promotion consistent with evidence on quality, safety and effectiveness, in line with patient choice and expectations. ③

分析：汉语句式中,尤其是在政治类的文献中,经常采用相同句式或短句,起到对偶或排比的效果,从而在修辞上对仗整齐,增加表达的气势。该汉语段落充分体现了这一特点。"提高收治率和治愈率、降低感染率和病亡率"是两组对照关系的动宾句式,"两提高、两降低""坚持……,坚持……",以及"集中……集中……集中……集中……"是非常明显的排比关系,起到增强表达效果的作用。对比英文句中,则以"member states should consider"的主谓结构为统辖,使用形容词短语"mindful of . . ." "consistent with . . ."、分词短语"including . . ."、介词短语"in line with . . ."等不同的

---

① 选自《大麻法案》第二部分"历史回顾"第二小节"二十世纪中期"第一段。
② 选自《抗击新冠》白皮书第二部分"防控和救治两个战场协同作战"第三小节"全力救治患者、拯救生命"第一段。
③ 选自《传统医学战略》第四部分"战略目标、战略方向和战略行动"中的第三个战略目标第四段。

语法结构与主句一起形成层级分明、句法结构严谨的复杂句。

二、段落翻译的特点和策略

1. 无主语句

对于汉语中的无主语句,需要根据语境的具体情况进行判断,采用不同的翻译方法。有些句子的主语隐含在上下文的语境中,可以通过在原文基础上添加必要的单词或词组等充当主语,使译文在语法和句式结构上符合英语中对主谓结构的要求。还可以调整句子结构,采用形式主语、祈使句、被动语态等形式进行翻译。

[例5] 随着人类的进化,开始有目的地寻找防治疾病的药物和方法,所谓"神农尝百草""药食同源",就是当时的真实写照。①

译文：As time went by, people began to actively seek out such remedies and methods for preventing and treating diseases. Sayings like "Shennong (Celestial Farmer) tasting a hundred herbs" and "food and medicine coming from the same source" are characteristic of those years.

分析：中文原句中,谓语动词"寻找"的逻辑主语应该是人们或者人类,因此在译文中增添了"people"这一主语,使译文符合英语语法的要求,同时将原文中的四个分句分为两句翻译,第二个句子中以"神农尝百草""药食同源"作为判断句的主语,这两句属于古代医学的格言,因此增加了"sayings"作为主语,将"神农尝百草""药食同源"处理为介词"like"的宾语。

[例6] ① 坚持中西医结合、中西药并用,② 发挥中医药治未病、辨证施治、多靶点干预的独特优势,全程参与深度介入疫情防控,③ 从中医角度研究确定病因病基、治则治法,④ 形成了覆盖医学观察期、轻型、普通型、重型、危重型、恢复期发病全过程的中医诊疗规范和技术方案,在全国范围内全面推广使用。②

译文：① Both TCM and Western medicine were used and traditional Chinese and Western drugs administered. ② China has leveraged the unique strength of TCM in preemptive prevention, differentiated medication, and multi-targeted intervention, and at every step of COVID-19 treatment and control. ③ The etiology and pathogen of the

---

① 选自《中国的中医药》白皮书第一部分"中医药的历史发展"第一小节"中医药历史发展脉络"第一段。

② 选自《抗击新冠》白皮书第二部分"防控和救治两个战场协同作战"第三小节"全力救治患者、拯救生命"第五段。

disease were analyzed and confirmed through TCM methodology, as were the principles and methods of treatment. ④ A set of TCM diagnosis and treatment protocols were developed to cover the entire process of medical observation, treatment of mild, moderate, severe, and critical cases, and recovery, and they have been applied nationwide.

分析：中文原句较长，含有多个动宾结构却没有明显的主语。在翻译时，译者将原句划分为 4 个英语句子，灵活运用主、被动语态，将原句中"坚持……，发挥……，参与……，确定……，形成……，全面推广……"6 个动宾结构分别用不同的策略进行处理。①句中"坚持……"使用被动语态译为"... were used"；②句中"发挥……，参与……"则进行合译，同时增添了逻辑主语"China"，以符合英语表达习惯；③、④句中"确定……，形成……"使用了被动语态，将"病因病基"和"中医诊疗规范和技术方案"作为主语置于句首，以突出信息。并且在第④句中，用"and"连接并列句，同样使用被动语态，以"they"做主语代指前文，保持信息的连贯性。

2. 连动句

英语句子要求以主谓结构为统辖，充分应用各种表示关系和连接的词汇，如介词（词组）、连词、关系代词（副词）、连接代词（副词）、非谓语动词等，形成显性衔接的多类型从句（孙中有，2022：48）。因此中文的连动长句在翻译时，可考虑拆分、合并等不同方法，根据原文语义进行切分，调整为若干英语主谓结构句型，并将原文逻辑关系显化，有效传达原文信息。

[例 7] ① 秦汉时期（前 221—公元 220）的中医典籍《黄帝内经》，② 系统论述了人的生理、病理、疾病以及"治未病"和疾病治疗的原则及方法，③ 确立了中医学的思维模式，④ 标志着从单纯的临床经验积累发展到了系统理论总结阶段，⑤ 形成了中医药理论体系框架。①

译文：①② *The Huang Di Nei Jing* (*Yellow Emperor's Inner Canon*) compiled during the Qin and Han times (221 BC – AD 220) offered systematic discourses on human physiology, on pathology, on the symptoms of illness, on preventative treatment, and on the principles and methods of treatment. ③④ This book defined the framework of TCM, thus serving as a landmark in TCM's development and symbolizing the

---

① 选自《中国的中医药》白皮书第一部分"中医药的历史发展"第一小节"中医药历史发展脉络"第一段。

transformation from the accumulation of clinical experience to the systematic summation of theories. ⑤ A theoretical framework for TCM had been in place.

分析： 中文原句共 5 个分句，以"《黄帝内经》"做主语，后接 4 个谓语动词，是一个典型的连动句。在翻译时，译者根据语义进行了切分，将前两个分句译为一句，并将"系统论述"后的一连串宾语译为并列的介词短语。将第三句和第四分句合译为一句，用"this book"做主语，代指"《黄帝内经》"，并且以第③分句为主谓结构，将第④分句处理为分词短语，且使用显性连接词"thus"来表现两个分句之间的逻辑关系。第⑤分句则以"a theoretical framework"做主语，突出了这一时期中医发展的主要成就，同时在句式结构上有了变化，避免了单一结构的单调重复，长短句相结合，节奏更加富于变化。

[例8] 医疗救治始终以提高收治率和治愈率、降低感染率和病亡率的"两提高""两降低"为目标，坚持集中患者、集中专家、集中资源、集中救治"四集中"原则，坚持中西医结合，实施分类救治、分级管理。

译文： From the outset, China's goal in its medical response to COVID-19 has been to improve the patient admission and cure rates and reduce the infection and fatality rates. The infected were treated in dedicated medical facilities where medical specialists from all over the country and all the necessary medical resources were concentrated. Both traditional Chinese medicine and Western medicine were applied. A condition-specific and category-based approach was applied to medical treatment of patients.

分析： 在翻译政治文献中的排比结构时，应根据具体语境，适当采用语义融合的翻译策略，不必保留原文中的"坚持……坚持……"，或"集中……集中……集中……集中……"排比结构，以免在英文中出现不必要的重复。此外，对于"两提高""两降低""四集中"这样的数字缩略语，英文中并没有对应的表达习惯，且原文中已包含其所指代的具体内容，翻译时应灵活处理，译出其具体所指内容，而不必对数字缩略语进行直译。

第四节 词语的翻译

《中国的中医药》《抗击新冠》等白皮书包含大量中医理论、中医著作及医家，以及中医治疗方法和原则等具有中医特色的文化负载词，在英译时需注意其词汇层面的不同特点,采用适当的翻译策略,在准确体现词汇内涵的同时提高受众的接受度。

一、文化负载词的翻译策略

文化负载词是标志某种文化中特有事物的词、词组和习语,反映了一个民族在漫长的历史进程中逐渐积累并与其他国家截然不同的独特活动方式(廖七一,2000:232)。中医文化是中华传统文化的组成部分,中医语言中有大量的文化负载词,承载丰富的中国古代哲学思想,具有浓厚的人文色彩。翻译文化负载词时,应根据情况对原文进行变通,采用增译、释译等方式灵活处理。

[**例 1**] 春秋战国(前 770—前 221)时期,扁鹊总结前人经验,提出"望、闻、问、切"四诊合参的方法,奠定了中医临床诊断和治疗的基础。①

译文:During the Spring and Autumn and Warring States Period (770 – 221 BC), Bian Que drew on the experience of his predecessors and put forward the four diagnostic methods—inspection, auscultation & olfaction, inquiry, and palpation, laying the foundation for TCM diagnosis and treatment.

分析:在翻译"望闻问切"四诊合参这一中医诊断学核心概念时,译者先明确"望、闻、问、切"均为诊断方法(diagnostic methods),再进一步说明其代表的具体内容。鉴于白皮书这一正式文体的特征,"闻诊"译为"auscultation & olfaction",而没有选择普通读者更易于接受和理解的"listening and smelling"。

[**例 2**] 同时期的《神农本草经》,概括论述了君臣佐使、七情合和、四气五味等药物配伍和药性理论……②

译文:The *Shen Nong Ben Cao Jing* (*Shennong's Classic of Materia Medica*)—another masterpiece of medical literature appeared during this period—outlines the theory of the compatibility of medicinal ingredients. For example, it holds that a prescription should include at the same time the jun (or sovereign), chen (or minister), zuo (or assistant) and shi (or messenger) ingredient drugs, and should give expression to the harmony of the seven emotions as well as the properties of drugs known as "four natures" and "five flavors."

分析:本句中,对《神农本草经》这一著作,译者采用了拼音加直译和增译的方

---

① 选自《中国的中医药》白皮书第一部分"中医药的历史发展"第一小节"中医药历史发展脉络"第一段。

② 同上。

式,便于缺乏汉语背景的外国读者更好地了解这部著作。"君臣佐使"是方剂配伍的基本原则,采用中医文化中常见的隐喻方式来说明中药处方中不同药物所起的不同作用。译者采用拼音加直译的方法,保留了该术语的文化和理论内涵,海外读者根据前面的概括词"the compatibility of medicinal ingredients"和后面的"ingredient drugs"类别词,可以更好地理解"君臣佐使"的含义。此处增译的"at the same time"似乎不妥,容易引起读者的误解,也并非原文之意,众所周知,中药配伍中并非所有的药方都同时包含君臣佐使这四种不同的成分。此外,"七情合和""四气五味"是对中医中药物配伍和药性分类的高度概括,译者将"四气五味"译为"the properties of drugs known as 'four natures' and 'five flavors'",在原文的基础上进行了词序的调整,使意义表达更为清晰。将"七情合和"译为"the harmony of the seven emotions",理解似乎有所偏差。译者将"七情"理解为内外因理论中的七种情志,但此处是指中医配伍中的七情合和,即中药配伍的七种不同作用——单行、相使、相须、相畏、相杀、相恶、相反的合称,用以说明中药配伍后药效、毒性变化的关系(陈德兴、张玉萍、徐丽莉等,2012:4),应译为"seven compatibility methods"(WHO 术语标准),或"seven relations of medicinal compatibility"(世界中医药学会联合会术语标准)。

[例3]　进入西周时期(前 1046—前 771),开始有了食医、疾医、疡医、兽医的分工。①

译文:In the Western Zhou Dynasty(1046－771 BC),doctors began to be classified into four categories—dietician, physician, doctor of decoctions and veterinarian.

分析:"食医、疾医、疡医、兽医"是周朝开始对医官的分类,在翻译时,译者将其译为与现代医学中大致对等的名称:dietician, physician, doctor of decoctions and veterinarian,让读者更容易理解其不同的含义。但是其中对"疡医"的理解有误,"疡医"一词始见于《周礼·天官》(陈成国点校,1989:12),"掌肿疡、溃疡、金疡、折疡之祝药劀杀之齐",即治疗肿疡、溃疡、金疮、折伤等外科疾患的医生,相当于外科医生,与"疾医"相对,世界中医药学会联合会术语标准将其翻译为"sore and wound doctor"。

二、积极、正面的国家/文化/中医形象的构建

中医药白皮书是中国政府向世界介绍中医药、促进中医药对外交流的宣传文

---

① 选自《中国的中医药》白皮书第一部分"中医药的历史发展"第一小节"中医药历史发展脉络"第一段。

本,目的是将中医药作为中国优秀传统文化的代表,向国外介绍中医药的特色和价值,提高国际社会对传统中医药的认可度和接受度。白皮书中需展现中医药积极、正面的形象,因此翻译时也要注意在词汇和修辞的选择上有助于实现这一目的(罗茜,2019:32)。

[例4]　同时期的《神农本草经》⋯⋯对于合理处方、安全用药、提高疗效具有十分重要的指导作用,为中药学理论体系的形成与发展奠定了基础。①

译文:All this provides guidance to the production of TCM prescriptions, safe application of TCM drugs and enhancement of the therapeutic effects, thus laying the foundation for the formation and development of TCM pharmaceutical theory.

分析:本句中着重强调了《神农本草经》在中药学方面的主要内容以及在中药学发展上的重要意义,其中"guidance""safe""enhancement""therapeutic effects"等词汇突出强调了中药在治疗方面的安全性及疗效,有力地凸显了中医药疗效显著且用药安全方面的独特优势。

[例5]　明代(1368—1644),李时珍的《本草纲目》,在世界上首次对药用植物进行了科学分类,创新发展了中药学的理论和实践,是一部药物学和博物学巨著。②

译文:A herbology and nature masterpiece, the *Ben Cao Gang Mu* (*Compendium of Materia Medica*) compiled by Li Shizhen in the Ming Dynasty (1368 – 1644) was the first book in the world that scientifically categorized medicinal herbs. It was a pioneering work that advanced TCM pharmaceutical theory.

分析:《本草纲目》是一部具有世界影响力的中国药学典籍,达尔文和李约瑟都曾在著作中引用此书,此书以纲带目、纲举目张的分类方式非常接近现代科学的认识,因此译文中用"scientifically categorized"来描述《本草纲目》的这一创新性的特点,非常贴切。《本草纲目》在植物学方面的研究处于当时的世界领先水平,具有重大的科学价值,因此译文中使用了"pioneering work"来概括《本草纲目》在中药发展史以及世界科学史上的重要地位。这些积极正面的词汇凸显出中医药的科学性和先进性,符合白皮书对外宣传和构建中医药正面积极形象的目的。

[例6]　关心关爱医务人员,制定一系列保障政策,开展心理疏导,妥善安排轮

---

①　选自《中国的中医药》白皮书第一部分"中医药的历史发展"第一小节"中医药历史发展脉络"第一段。

②　同上。

换休整,缓解身体和心理压力,保持一线医务人员战斗力。①

译文:Health workers have been cared for and their needs attended to. A series of policies and measures have been introduced to ensure their wellbeing, such as psychological counseling and staff rotation, to ease their physical and psychological stress, help them stay healthy, and allow them to continue the fight on the front line.

分析:本句主要关于抗击疫情中对医务人员的关爱,因此在译文中,除了用"cared for ... needs attended to"翻译"关心关爱医务人员"外,还增译了"to ensure their wellbeing""help them stay healthy",以突出对医务人员健康的关注,向国际社会展现抗疫中的人文关怀,让抗疫不仅有力度,而且有温度。

此外,在《抗击新冠》白皮书中,大量使用到了隐喻表达。据统计,白皮书的隐喻类型可以分为9类,如战争类、人体类、自然类、建筑类等(辛红娟、严文钏,2022:80-81),其中战争相关的隐喻最多,如"打响抗击疫情的人民战争、总体战、阻击战""医务工作者白衣执甲、逆行出征",将防控疫情的严峻形势比喻为战争,将医务工作者比喻为身披白衣的战士。使用战争类的隐喻将疫情喻为威胁生命安全的敌人,能够凸显抗疫的艰巨性和严峻性,强调我国为取得抗疫胜利付出的艰辛努力,以及战胜疫情的坚定斗志(冯正斌、刘振清,2022:70)。而且,白皮书以战争隐喻为实现逻辑衔接的连贯工具,将全文紧密衔接,提高了语篇的连贯性。本例中"保持一线医务人员战斗力"便是沿用此类战争隐喻,译者将其意译为"allow them to continue the fight on the front line",即确保医务人员能战斗在一线,表现出医务工作者奋战一线、守护健康、英勇无畏的精神。

要注意的是,对于原文中的战争隐喻不可一概而论,全部进行直译。适当使用战争隐喻有助于构筑良好的国家形象,表现中国政府和人民团结一心、严肃认真对待"疫情战争"的态度,但滥用战争隐喻和"战式表达"则会给国际读者造成文化冲突感,留下中国好战、侵略的不良形象,因此需要谨慎使用。例如,《抗击新冠》原文中的"国有企业发挥主力军作用……",译文处理为"State-owned enterprises have taken the lead in ... ",用"take the lead"来翻译"主力军",保留了原文的意义,而消除了战争隐喻的形式。

三、汉语行文中的冗余重复表达

汉语在行文中善用四字格词,读起来节奏感强,对仗工整,能够增强表达效果,且

---

① 选自《抗击新冠》白皮书第二部分"防控和救治两个战场协同作战"第三小节"全力救治患者、拯救生命"第七段。

汉语中还往往使用一些华丽的辞藻,显得文采飞扬,具有感染力。但是在翻译时,一方面很难找到与中文四字格词形式对等的英文表达,另一方面,有些表达在意义上是有重叠和交叉的,或者并没有太多的实际意义,完全直译则会让外国读者感觉重复拉杂,反而冲淡表达效果,降低译文的接受度。翻译时需要根据国外受众的思维习惯,对中文原文进行适当加工,灵活运用不同的翻译策略,以达到理想的翻译效果。

[例7] 唐代(618—907),孙思邈提出的"大医精诚",体现了中医对医道精微、心怀至诚、言行诚谨的追求,是中华民族高尚的道德情操和卓越的文明智慧在中医药中的集中体现,是中医药文化的核心价值理念。①

译文:Sun Simiao, a great doctor of the Tang Dynasty (618 - 907), proposed that mastership of medicine lies in proficient medical skills and lofty medical ethics, which eventually became the embodiment of a moral value of the Chinese nation, a core value that has been conscientiously upheld by the TCM circles.

分析:原文中连续使用了"大医精诚""医道精微""心怀至诚""言行诚谨"等四字格词,以及"中华民族高尚的道德情操和卓越的文明智慧"这样的溢美之词,让中国读者能够明显感受到中医药对医学道德伦理的推崇,极大地提升自豪感和自信心。但如果按照原文逐字翻译,则难免有词藻堆砌之感,反而显得过于夸张而不真实,因此译者进行了较多的整合调整。"大医精诚"一词虽然简洁,却内涵丰富,是指优秀的医生不仅要医术精湛,还应具有高尚的医德,因此译者在此处进行了释译,突出强调了"proficient medical skills and lofty medical ethics",抓住了"大医精诚"一词的核心内涵,而"医道精微""心怀至诚""言行诚谨"均是对"大医精诚"的诠释,译文进行了删减,以避免重复。后一句"是中华民族高尚的道德情操和卓越的文明智慧在中医药中的集中体现"也进行了简化,以"the embodiment of a moral value of the Chinese nation"进行概括,信息更加直接明确,避免产生语义重复,造成结构上的冗余,从而符合英语阅读者的阅读习惯。

[例8] 武汉市针对患者数量急剧增长、80%左右是轻症的情况,集中力量将一批体育场馆、会展中心等改造成16家方舱医院,床位达到1.4万余张,使轻症患者应收尽收、应治尽治,减少了社区感染传播,减少了轻症向重症转化。②

---

① 选自《中国的中医药》白皮书第一部分"中医药的历史发展"第一小节"中医药历史发展脉络"第一段。

② 选自《抗击新冠》白皮书第二部分"防控和救治两个战场协同作战"第三小节"全力救治患者、拯救生命"第三段。

译文：In Wuhan, faced with surging infections and considering that 80 percent of cases were mild, the city government mobilized resources to repurpose stadiums and exhibition centers into 16 temporary treatment centers. With some 14,000 beds, these centers were able to admit all confirmed mild cases for treatment. This helped to reduce infections and virus transmission in communities and prevent mild cases from worsening.

分析：原文后半句中的"应收尽收、应治尽治"是政府文书中常见到的四字结构，在中文中可以显得结构整齐，句式统一。在翻译时可采用直译的形式，将四字结构的含义译出，而不必追求形式上的节奏感。最后的两个排比结构"减少……，减少……"的译文，译出的是其中的内容含义，而不必保留形式上的一致。

第五节　翻译练习与任务

一、翻译练习

1. 下列术语选自《中国的中医药》等政府文书，请将中文译为英文。

（1）治未病

（2）因人、因时、因地制宜

（3）道法自然，天人合一

（4）中西医并重

（5）扶持中医药和民族医药事业发展

（6）国务院联防联控机制

（7）国家中医药管理局

（8）重大突发公共卫生事件一、二、三级响应

（9）清肺排毒汤

（10）社区传播和聚集性传播案例

2. 请将下列句子译为英文，注意对比中英文句式结构的不同，并运用适当的翻译策略进行调整。

（1）中医强调生活方式和健康有着紧密关系，主张以养生为要务，认为可通过情志调摄、劳逸适度、膳食合理、起居有常等，也可根据不同体质或状态给予适当干预，以养神健体，培育正气，提高抗邪能力，从而达到保健和防病作用。

（2）中医药已成为中国与东盟、欧盟、非洲、中东欧等组织和地区卫生经贸合作的重要内容，成为中国与世界各国开展人文交流、促进东西方文明交流互鉴的重要内容，成为中国与各国共同维护世界和平、增进人类福祉、建设人类命运共同体的重要载体。

（3）中国将学习借鉴各种现代文明成果，坚持古为今用，推进中医药现代化，切实把中医药继承好、发展好、利用好，努力实现中医药健康养生文化的创造性转化、创新性发展，使之与现代健康理念相融相通，服务于人民健康，服务于健康中国建设。

（4）中共中央总书记、国家主席、中央军委主席习近平赴湖北省武汉市考察疫情防控工作，指出经过艰苦努力，湖北和武汉疫情防控形势发生积极向好变化，取得阶段性重要成果，但疫情防控任务依然艰巨繁重，要慎终如始、再接再厉、善作善成，坚决打赢湖北保卫战、武汉保卫战。

（5）一方有难，八方支援。疫情发生后，全国上下紧急行动，依托强大综合国力，开展全方位的人力组织战、物资保障战、科技突击战、资源运动战，全力支援湖北省和武汉市抗击疫情，在最短时间集中最大力量阻断疫情传播。

（6）在中央指导组指导下，武汉市部署实施确诊患者、疑似患者、发热患者、确诊患者的密切接触者"四类人员"分类集中管理，按照应收尽收、应治尽治、应检尽检、应隔尽隔"四应"要求，持续开展拉网排查、集中收治、清底排查三场攻坚战。

二、翻译任务

以下段落分别选自 2016 年 12 月颁布的《中华人民共和国中医药法》和中国针灸学会 2020 年 3 月印发的《新型冠状病毒肺炎针灸干预的指导意见（第二版）》。请以小组形式选择其中一个段落进行翻译。要求根据汉英文本在语篇、段落及词汇层面的不同特点，采用适当的翻译策略，并体会如何通过不同的翻译策略，提高译文的接受度，树立积极正面的国家形象。

（1）中医药，是包括汉族和少数民族医药在内的我国各民族医药的统称，是反映中华民族对生命、健康和疾病的认识，具有悠久历史传统和独特理论及技术方法的医药学体系。

中医药事业是我国医药卫生事业的重要组成部分。国家大力发展中医药事业，实行中西医并重的方针，建立符合中医药特点的管理制度，充分发挥中医药在我国医药卫生事业中的作用。

发展中医药事业应当遵循中医药发展规律，坚持继承和创新相结合，保持和发挥中医药特色和优势,运用现代科学技术,促进中医药理论和实践的发展。国家鼓励中医西医相互学习,相互补充,协调发展,发挥各自优势,促进中西医结合。

(2)新冠肺炎属中医"疫"病范畴。数千年来,中医学在长期与疫病作斗争的医疗实践中,积累了丰富的经验。针灸是中医学重要组成部分,并具有自身鲜明特色和独特优势,在我国抗疫历史上做出了重要贡献。我国古典医籍有针灸防疫治病的相关记载。如唐代医家孙思邈在《备急千金要方》提出:"凡人吴蜀地游官,体上常须三两处灸之,勿令疮暂差,则瘴疬温疟毒气不能著人也。"明代医家李时珍在《本草纲目》阐述:"艾叶……。灸之则透诸经而治百种病邪,起沉疴之人为康泰,其功亦大矣。"均载明针灸可以预防和治疗传染病。现代临床和实验研究表明,针灸可调节人体免疫功能,具有抗炎、抗感染的作用,在传染病的防治中起到了较好作用。面对突如其来的新冠肺炎,中医针灸积极参与防治已取得较好的效果。随着对新冠肺炎认识的深入和中医针灸诊疗经验的积累,根据国家卫生健康委员会办公厅、国家中医药管理局办公厅印发的《新型冠状病毒肺炎诊疗方案(试行第六版)》以及《新型冠状病毒肺炎恢复期中医康复指导建议(试行)》,我们形成了《新型冠状病毒肺炎针灸干预的指导意见(第二版)》,供医务工作者在针灸实施与指导居家患者时参阅。

三、扩展阅读

[1]罗茜.评价系统视角下中医形象构建的话语策略研究——以《中国的中医药》白皮书英译本为例[J].中医文献杂志,2019,37(6):32-36.

[2]辛红娟,严文钏.关联理论视角下的隐喻翻译研究——以《抗击新冠肺炎疫情的中国行动》英译为例[J].宁波大学学报(人文科学版),2022,35(4):79-84.

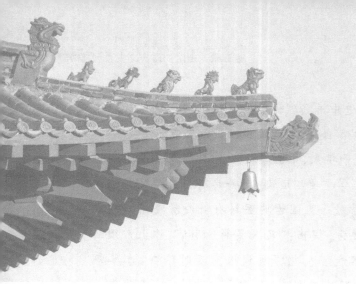

第三章
中医药新闻译写

有关中医药的新闻是中医药文化形象建构的重要载体之一,对提升国际中医药话语权发挥着重要作用。对外英语新闻报道是一种跨国家、跨文化、跨语言的传播。它的读者对象主要是使用英语阅读的外国人士,其根本任务是全面完整地反映中国政府的对内对外政策,客观反映中国在国际社会的形象,为国家的发展建设创造良好的国际环境。由于读者兴趣不同,价值观念不同,要实现不同文化互通,促进不同文明互鉴,不仅要让受众听得见、听得清,更要让他们听得懂、听得进。在对外翻译新闻之前,应有的放矢,提高报道内容对受众的针对性、接近性及适应性,以达到更好的传播效果。因此,对外英语新闻报道并非逐字对译,新闻英译要求清晰易懂(张健,2016:171-175)。倘若将有关新闻逐字逐句译成英文,势必影响传播效果。

第一节　语　料　导　入

本节的分析语料分为两组。第一组为汉语新闻报道,共 5 篇,分别选自央广网、新华网、喀麦隆资讯、中国日报网和上海中医药大学官网。第二组为与第一组相同主题内容的平行英语新闻报道,也共 5 篇,分别选自 CNN、*China Daily* 以及上海市人民政府网。10 篇新闻均公开发表于 2020 年至 2022 年间。语料涉及的五个主题依次为"三种治疗新冠肺炎的中药颗粒获批上市""中医药服务'一带一路'沿线人民健康""中国医疗队为喀麦隆贫困群众提供免费救治""中医药防治新冠肺炎发挥了哪些作用""上海中医药大学举办第二届'中医汉语桥'"。文中只对新闻标题、导语、主体文字部分进行语料分析,而忽略新闻图片说明等其他部分。

一、中文语料

1.《三种治疗新冠肺炎的中药颗粒获批上市》①

央广网北京3月3日消息(记者 宋雪)日前,国家药品监督管理局通过特别审批程序应急批准中国中医科学院中医临床基础医学研究所的清肺排毒颗粒、广东一方制药有限公司的化湿败毒颗粒、山东步长制药股份有限公司的宣肺败毒颗粒上市。

记者从国家药监局了解到,清肺排毒颗粒、化湿败毒颗粒、宣肺败毒颗粒是在武汉抗疫临床一线众多院士专家筛选出有效方药清肺排毒汤、化湿败毒方、宣肺败毒方的成果转化,均来源于古代经典名方,也是中药注册分类改革后首次按照《中药注册分类及申报资料要求》(2020年第68号)"3.2类　其他来源于古代经典名方的中药复方制剂"审评审批的品种。

清肺排毒颗粒用于感受寒湿疫毒所致的疫病,化湿败毒颗粒用于湿毒侵肺所致的疫病,宣肺败毒颗粒用于湿毒郁肺所致的疫病。

此前,在国家卫健委和国家中医药管理局联合印发的数版新冠肺炎诊疗方案中,连花清瘟胶囊(颗粒)与金花清感颗粒、疏风解毒胶囊(颗粒)等一批中成药屡次被推荐用于新冠肺炎临床治疗。清肺排毒颗粒、化湿败毒颗粒、宣肺败毒颗粒的上市将为新冠肺炎的治疗提供更多选择。

2.《中医药服务"一带一路"沿线人民健康》②

新华社北京9月3日电(记者高春霄、罗鑫、林苗苗)随着近年来中国推进中医药产业发展与合作、加快中医药"走出去"步伐,中医药越来越多地服务"一带一路"沿线国家和地区的人民。

作为2022年中国国际服务贸易交易会期间举办的论坛之一,第五届"一带一路"中医药发展论坛2日以线上线下结合的方式举行。中国国家中医药管理局局长于文明在致辞中说,中医药已传播至196个国家和地区,成为中国与东盟、欧盟、非盟以及上合组织、金砖国家等地区和组织合作的重要领域。

---

① 来源:央广网 https://baijiahao.baidu.com/s?id=1693189893078190371&wfr=spider&for=pc,搜索日期:2023 - 02 - 27。

② 来源:新华网 http://www.news.cn/politics/2022-09/03/c_1128972949.htm,搜索日期:2023 - 02 - 27。

2016年,北京中医药大学圣彼得堡中医中心在俄罗斯第二大城市圣彼得堡正式成立。该中心负责人、北京中医药大学教授刘清国对记者说,近年来俄罗斯民众对中医药的兴趣与日俱增,中医成为不少当地患者治疗方案的新选择。

"特别是在对包括颈椎病、腰椎病、神经性头痛等慢性病的治疗和康复中,中医药疗效独特。"刘清国说,"一些患者开始只是抱着试一试的态度来尝试中医,后来疗效不错,经过口口相传,来中心看病的俄罗斯患者越来越多,还有来自白俄罗斯、意大利、荷兰等其他欧洲国家的患者。"

在常规临床治疗外,刘清国和其他中医还会给外国患者介绍中医理念,带他们到中医中心开设的练功房练气功、打太极拳。

自成立以来,北京中医药大学圣彼得堡中医中心为当地医生开设培训班,与当地医院定期开展学术交流,在当地开展义诊活动等。在刘清国看来,中医中心帮助俄罗斯民众了解中医药文化,成为外国人感知中国传统文化的一扇窗口。

近年来,中医药在越来越多"一带一路"沿线国家和地区"生根发芽"。在本届服贸会健康卫生服务专题展上,陕西中医药展团展示了首批国家中医药服务出口基地——西安中医脑病医院的最新成果。

2021年,西安中医脑病医院与哈萨克斯坦阿斯塔纳医科大学、纳扎尔巴耶夫大学医学院三方联建的西安国际脑病康复中心在哈萨克斯坦首都努尔苏丹正式开诊。目前共有3 700余人次前往就医。

西安中医脑病医院院长宋虎杰说:"中医诊疗技术在'一带一路'沿线国家和地区得到持续推广,中医药服务出口不断扩大,体现了这些国家和地区广大民众对中医药的信任。"

中医药交流合作已成为共建"一带一路"高质量发展的新亮点。2022年1月发布的《推进中医药高质量融入共建"一带一路"发展规划(2021—2025年)》提出,"十四五"时期,中国将与共建"一带一路"国家合作建设30个高质量中医药海外中心。

"'一带一路'沿线对于中医药'走出去'是一片广阔的天地。未来,中医药在这些国家和地区将有非常好的发展前景。"刘清国说。

3.《中国医疗队为喀麦隆贫困群众提供免费救治》①

周六,喀麦隆中部地区靠近首都雅温得的一个村庄体验到了幸福,因为中国医疗

---

① 来源:喀麦隆资讯 http://lmny. 52hrtt. com/cn/n/w/info/G1661309547000,搜索日期:2023 - 02 - 27。

队为居民提供了免费医疗服务。

据了解,Ngat-Bane 村周六接待了不同领域的中国医生来访。他们是来自超声、口腔、针灸等各个科室的 12 人。据报道,驻扎在雅温得市郊约 40 公里的姆巴尔马约镇的中国医疗队将前往 Ngat-Bane 卫生中心,为该地区民众免费提供医疗服务。

这一人道主义行动吸引了数十人前来就诊。来自附近村庄的 63 岁的理查德·梅科加(Richard Mekoga)称,他患有背痛、眼睛和神经问题。"这是我第一次参加(中国)健康运动。我对我们收到的方式非常满意,"梅科加说。该男子强调,他确信中国医疗队提供的药物能救他。

其他几名到访并接受采访的村民也是如此。请注意,Ngat-Bane 村与该地区的大多数村庄一样位于内陆地区,拥有丰富的野生动物和散落的茅草屋顶小屋。尽管这个地区生活着许多村民①,但没有医院,村民们负担不起在 Mbalmayo 医院寻求治疗。作为活动的一部分,中国医疗队捐赠了医疗物资。

4.《中医药防治新冠肺炎发挥了哪些作用?》②

国务院新闻办公室 3 月 23 日下午在湖北武汉举行新闻发布会,中西医专家介绍了中医药防治新冠肺炎的重要作用及有效药物。

中医药局党组书记余艳红介绍,全国新冠肺炎确诊病例中有 74 187 人使用了中医药,占 91.5%。从临床疗效观察来看,中医药总有效率达 90% 以上。

余艳红表示,中医药能够有效缓解症状;能够减少轻型普通型向重型发展;能够提高治愈率、降低病亡率;能够促进患者康复。

中国工程院院士黄璐琦研究员说,临床显示,宣肺败毒方在对照观察中可将淋巴细胞恢复率提高 17%,临床治愈率提高 22%。

北京中医医院院长刘清泉教授说,已经显示出金花清感和连花清瘟这两个药,临床上治疗新冠肺炎的轻型和普通型还是有非常确切的疗效的,血必净注射液针对炎症风暴、凝血功能紊乱等治疗也有很好的疗效。

中国工程院院士张伯礼教授说,中医的方舱医院中,564 名患者没有一例转为重症的。取得经验以后,向别的方舱也推广,一万多名患者普遍使用了中药。方舱中医综合治疗,显著降低了由轻症转为重症的比例。

中国工程院院士、中国中医科学院院长黄璐琦认为,中医和西医虽属于两个不

---

① 原文使用了"灵魂"一词,疑为英文中"soul"一词的误译,这里将"灵魂"改为"村民"。

② 来源:https://language.chinadaily.com.cn/a/202003/24/WS5e798065a31012282172818db.html,搜索日期:2023 - 02 - 27。

同的医学体系,对健康、疾病有不同的认识角度,但是它们都会基于临床疗效这一事实。

余艳红表示,这次的实践再次充分证明,中医药学这个老祖宗留下来的宝贵财富依然好使、管用,并且经济易行。我们愿意与所有国家分享宝贵经验及有效治疗手段。

5.《结缘中医·上中医举办第二届"中医汉语桥"》①

11月18日,第二届"中医汉语桥"在上海中医药大学国际教育学院举办,动人的校园秋色迎来了一批新、老朋友。

来自印度的Harsha已经是第二次报名"中医汉语桥"了,去年的活动把她从"汉语迷"变成了"中医爱好者"。来自日本的森田未央、高桥美树、沟上阳子与中医的结缘也是从上中医的汉语课堂开始的,目前她们已是汉语言(中医药方向)本科一年级新生,汉语带她们认识了中国,中医行业成了她们的职业选择。

"中医汉语桥"以目见、耳闻、身经体察等方式,引导外国友人学会观察日常生活中无处不在的中医文化。上中医外语教学中心的金静老师"一问、二听、三讨论",与外国友人探讨了啃秋、晒秋、贴秋膘等节气风俗蕴含的中医智慧,围绕"节气、习俗、药膳",送来了一份秋日节气养生攻略,让源于生活的中医应用于生活。

"雷氏"藿香香牌手作体验课程传播了"闻香防病、强身健体"的理念。藿香、丁香、薄荷研磨成粉,香粉揉捏成团,芳香萦绕指尖,疗愈身心。

不同汉语水平的外国友人走进了初、中、高级汉语课堂。在初级课堂掌握生存汉语,在中级课堂夯实语法基础,在高级课堂挑战成语文化,学员们展现了学习汉语和中国文化的浓厚兴趣。

汉语和中医具有相同的文化脉络,是中华民族两张最亮丽的文化名片。"中医汉语桥"以汉语为媒、文化筑桥,为外国友人提供了一个了解中医、实践汉语的平台。

二、英文语料

1. China Approves Sale of Traditional Medicine Products to Treat COVID-19 (《中国批准三种治疗新冠肺炎的中药上市》)②

CNN—China has approved three traditional Chinese medicine (TCM) products for

---

① 来源:https://www. shutcm. edu. cn/2022/1121/c205a147148/page. htm,搜索日期:2023 - 02 - 27。

② 来源:CNN App,搜索日期:2023 - 02 - 27。

sale to help treat COVID-19, the government's National Medical Products Administration announced on Wednesday.

The agency used a special approval procedure to green-light the three products, which "provide more options for COVID-19 treatment," it said in a statement.

The herbal products come in granular form and trace their origins to "ancient Chinese prescriptions," said the statement. They were developed from TCM remedies that had been used early in the pandemic, and that were "screened by many academics and experts on the front line."

The three products are "lung-clearing and detoxing granules" "dampness-resolving and detoxing granules", and "lung-diffusing and detoxing granules", said the statement.

2. China Focus：TCM Gains Popularity Among Belt and Road Countries(《中国焦点：中医药在"一带一路"国家越来越受欢迎》)①

BEIJING—Traditional Chinese Medicine has become a new option for patients in countries along the Belt and Road, amid China's promotion of TCM overseas and endeavors at TCM development and cooperation in recent years.

Yu Wenming, head of the National Administration of Traditional Chinese Medicine (NATCM), said on Friday that TCM has evolved into a significant international collaboration field and expanded to 196 countries and regions. Yu delivered his comments at the fifth Belt and Road Forum for TCM Development, a themed forum of the 2022 China International Fair for Trade in Services.

In recent years, Russian people's interest in TCM has increased, and TCM has become a new treatment option for many local patients, according to Liu Qingguo, a professor from Beijing University of Chinese Medicine and head of a TCM center in St. Petersburg, Russia. Established in 2016, the Russian center is affiliated to BUCM.

"TCM has unique curative effects for chronic diseases, such as spondylosis and tension-type headache," said Liu. "Our patients started by trying out the medicine, and later more Russians and even people from Belarus, Italy and other European countries, came for treatment as the center had established a reputation."

---

① 来源：China Daily https：//www. chinadaily. com. cn/a/202209/04/WS6314b629a310fd2b29e75 d2f. html,搜索日期：2023－02－27。

As more patients developed their interest in TCM culture, Liu and his colleagues showed them Qigong and Tai Chi in the center's practice room. These traditional Chinese martial arts focus on exploiting the human body's inner energy to achieve physical and mental harmony.

In addition to routine therapy, the TCM center has also conducted academic exchanges with local hospitals and organized training programs for local doctors, according to Liu.

China has also teamed up with other Belt and Road countries on TCM to tackle illnesses, as shown by the exhibitors at CIFTIS.

In 2021, Xi'an TCM Hospital of Encephalopathy in northwest China's Shaanxi Province, Astana Medical University and the School of Medicine of Nazarbayev University jointly set up a rehabilitation center for brain diseases at Nur-Sultan, the capital of Kazakhstan. Over 3,700 people have sought treatment at the center.

"The growing popularity of TCM treatment technologies and the expanding trade in services of TCM indicate that people in Belt and Road countries have confidence in TCM," said Song Hujie, president of the hospital.

During the 14th Five-Year Plan period (2021－2025), China aims to jointly establish 30 high-quality TCM centers with countries along the Belt and Road, according to a plan issued by central government agencies, including the NATCM, in January.

Chen Zhu, vice chairman of the National People's Congress Standing Committee, said China is ready to work with Belt and Road countries to promote the preservation and innovation of TCM, enhance its role in combating the COVID-19 pandemic and jointly build a global community of health for all.

3. Chinese Medical Team Provides Free Health Care Services in Rural Cameroon(《中国医疗队在喀麦隆农村提供免费医疗服务》)①

YAOUNDE—A Chinese medical team in Cameroon on Saturday provided free medical services to the people of Ngat-Bane, a village in the Centre region where the capital, Yaounde is located.

---

① 来源：China Daily https：//global. chinadaily. com. cn/a/202208/21/WS63021389a310fd2b29e 7362f_1. html,搜索日期：2023－02－27。

Early in the morning, more than one hundred villagers gathered in the Health Center of Ngat-Bane to welcome 12 doctors from various departments of ultrasound, stomatology, acupuncture, etc. of the Chinese medical team based in Mbalmayo, a town located about 40 km on the outskirts of Yaounde.

Among them was 63-year-old Richard Mekoga who came from a neighboring village. Mekoga said he was suffering from back pain and eye and nerve problems.

"This is my first time participating in the (Chinese) health campaign. I was extremely satisfied with how we were received," Mekoga said, adding that he was certain the medicine provided by the Chinese medical team will save him.

Ngat-Bane, like many other Cameroonian villages, has abundant wildlife and dispersed thatched huts, but zero hospitals. Villagers are often troubled by such health problems as rheumatism, typhoid, and malaria, but most of them cannot afford medical services in Mbalmayo.

"It (Chinese free consultation and treatment) relieves us, we who don't have enough means and who can't even travel to Mbalmayo (for treatment)," said 70-year-old Joseph Mbede Onambele who had been suffering from inflammation in the limbs and sometimes travels to Mbalmayo to receive medical treatment from Chinese health workers who work there.

Dieudonne Zang Mba Obele, mayor of Mbalmayo estimated that 70 percent of those who consulted and were treated free of charge were women and children.

"I believe this is an example of cooperation (between Cameroon and China). They (Chinese health workers) are not only for the district hospital of Mbalmayo but for the poorest populations who cannot go to the hospital of Mbalmayo, sometimes for lack of means, lack of infrastructure," Obele said.

As part of the campaign, the Chinese medical team donated medical supplies.

4. 原文无标题①

On the afternoon of March 23, the Information Office of the State Council held a press conference in Wuhan, Hubei Province. Experts of traditional Chinese medicine and

Western medicine introduced the important role and effective drugs of traditional Chinese medicine in preventing and treating COVID-19.

A total of 74, 187 confirmed patients, which account for 91. 5 percent of the total infections on the Chinese mainland, have been administered traditional Chinese medicine (TCM) as part of their treatment, and over 90 percent of them have shown improvement during clinical observation, according to Yu Yanhong, Party secretary and top official of the National Administration of Traditional Chinese Medicine.

TCM has effectively relieved symptoms, cut the rate of patients developing into severe conditions, raised the recovery rate, reduced the mortality rate and boosted patients' recovery, Yu said.

XuanFeiBaiDu Granule can increase the lymphocyte recovery rate by 17 percent and the clinical cure rate by 22 percent in the controlled observation, according to Huang Luqi, an academician of the Chinese Academy of Engineering.

Liu Qingquan, head of the Beijing Hospital of Traditional Chinese Medicine, said that two TCM drugs—Jinhua Qinggan Granule and Lianhua Qingwen Capsule / Granule have proven to be effective in the treatment of mild COVID-19 cases, while Xuebijing Injection can help treat inflammation and coagulation dysfunction.

Zhang Boli, an academician of the Chinese Academy of Engineering, said that TCM treatment has significantly lowered the proportion of patients whose conditions turned from mild to severe. "None of the 564 patients at the TCM-oriented temporary hospital in Wuhan saw their health condition deteriorating into severe," said Zhang. "We have therefore applied TCM treatment to over 10, 000 patients in other makeshift hospitals, and the rate of patients developing into severe conditions were substantially reduced," said Zhang.

TCM and Western medicine may come from two different medical systems and have different perspectives on health and diseases, but they are both based on the standard of factual clinical efficacy.

The practice of treating COVID-19 patients has proved once again that the precious wisdom left by our TCM ancestors is still practical, effective and economical. We would love to share these valuable experiences and effective treatment methods with all countries.

5. Second "TCM Chinese Bridge" Program Opens in Shanghai(《第二届"中医汉语桥"在上海开幕》)①

Shanghai University of Traditional Chinese Medicine (TCM) held the second "TCM Chinese Bridge" Program on campus on Nov 18, offering foreigners a fast track for Chinese language and medicine learning.

Among the foreign participants, Harsha Niraj from India signed up for the program for the second time. Last year's event turned her from a "Chinese language fan" to a "TCM enthusiast".

Three Japanese freshmen studying Chinese language at the university also participated in the program. Their interest in TCM began in their Chinese classes and now the TCM industry is expected to become their career choice.

The program aims to guide foreigners to learn how to observe the ubiquitous Chinese medicine culture in daily life by seeing, hearing and experiencing it.

Jin Jing, a teacher from the university's language teaching center, explained the wisdom behind Chinese medicine to the foreign participants, which can be learned through customs like fleshing out in autumn.

Jin also taught them how to stay healthy in autumn through a regimen that revolves around "solar terms, customs, and herbal cuisine".

The students also learned about smelling fragrances to prevent diseases and strengthen the body during a handmade sachet experience course.

Elementary, intermediate and advanced Chinese classes were also arranged for the foreigners according to their Chinese skills, and students demonstrated their strong interest in learning Chinese language and culture in the classes.

The two most precious cultural name cards of the Chinese people are Chinese language and Chinese medicine, both of which share the same cultural framework. The "TCM Chinese Bridge" Program uses Chinese language and culture as the medium to build bridges, providing a platform for foreigners to understand Chinese medicine and practice Chinese language.

---

① 来源：http://study.edu.sh.gov.cn/en/nc/news/2022-11-22/10163.html,搜索日期：2023 - 02 - 27。

第二节 篇 章 的 翻 译

一、英语新闻的基本结构

1. 纲要式结构

生活中,我们从报纸、杂志、广播、电视、网络等媒介都可获得各类新闻,有国际新闻、国内新闻,也有地方新闻。新闻内容包罗万象:政治、经济、科技、法律、军事、文娱、体育、灾难、暴力与犯罪、天气等等。新闻按事件的性质,可分为题材较严肃、侧重客观事实报道且具有一定时新性的硬新闻,以及人情味较浓、写法轻松活泼的软新闻。尽管新闻种类繁多,分类标准各异,但都必须通过记者按照不同的报道形式即新闻体裁予以采写。常见的新闻体裁主要有三类:消息(news)、特写(features)和新闻评论(commentaries and columns)。

本章内容收集的新闻语料主要来源于狭义的新闻,也就是纯消息报道,是突出新闻事实与时效性的硬新闻,也是最常用的新闻体裁。新闻消息通常主要由 3 个部分组成,即标题(headline)、导语(lead)和主体正文(body)。消息的基本结构最为常见的是倒金字塔结构(inverted pyramid form),按照重要性递减的顺序来报道新闻中的各项事实,最重要的信息最先报道,后面排列的新闻事实的重要程度、相关程度依次递减,因结构酷似一座倒置的金字塔而得名。

从上一节的 10 篇新闻语料来看,无论是汉语新闻还是英语新闻,无一例外都采用了倒金字塔结构。这一结构逐渐发展成为一种通用的国际惯例,其原因在于它具有以下优点:便于记者组织新闻材料和写作、便于编辑进行编改和剪辑、便于读者取舍并高效获取重要信息。

和其他类型的语篇一样,标题是新闻的中心思想,是全篇的题眼,也是导语的凝练和浓缩。标题通常会以更大的字体加黑印刷,以方便读者阅读抓取关键信息,帮助读者迅速决定是否要完整阅读该新闻。

新闻的第一段多为导语,开宗明义,开门见山。它是新闻最重要的组成部分,通常包含新闻六要素中的全部或几个要素,即5W1H:Who、What、When、Where、Why以及 How,写出最重要、最新鲜的资讯,回答人们普遍最关心的问题。

导语之后的新闻主体正文主要由众多新闻事实组成,通常分为多个小自然段,重要性由强至弱,每段报道一条新闻事实。为加强新闻的真实性和可读性,同时也为了方便读者理解新闻事件的内涵,相较于其他体裁,新闻还较多地使用直接引语或间接引语,提供一些必要的背景文字材料和解释。

下面分别以导入语料中汉语报道的第一篇和英语报道的第一篇为例,简要进行纲要式结构分析。两篇新闻消息是中美两国不同媒体对同一中医药新闻事件的报道,报道时间前后相隔一天。

《三种治疗新冠肺炎的中药颗粒获批上市》这篇消息从结构上而言,是一篇典型的倒金字塔结构消息。首先,标题部分言简意赅地介绍了全篇消息的新闻内容,并且因为加大加粗的字体而显得醒目、重要。紧接着,新闻电头"央广网北京3月3日消息"点明了消息的来源、报道媒体以及日期。其次,第一段作为导语,集中概括了"清肺排毒颗粒""化湿败毒颗粒"和"宣肺败毒颗粒"三种中药颗粒获国家药品监督管理局特别审批应急批准上市的消息。这一振奋人心的消息一下子抓住了读者的注意力,主要新闻要素得以清晰地呈现。再次,第二、三、四自然段按照新闻内容重要性递减的顺序对导语提示过的要点进行了补充和详述,先后交代了这三种中药颗粒在武汉抗疫实践中得到的检验和经方来源、它们各自适用的疾病类型,以及此前在新冠诊疗方案中被获批推荐使用的其他中药颗粒(胶囊)。

"China Approves sale of Traditional Medicine Products to Treat COVID-19"这篇消息从结构上而言,同样是一篇非常典型的倒金字塔结构消息。首先,标题部分简明扼要地概括了全篇消息的关键内容。标题字体加黑,处于最醒目的位置,夺人眼球。其次,第一自然段用一个句子"China has approved three traditional Chinese medicine (TCM) products for sale to help treat COVID-19, the government's National Medical Products Administration announced on Wednesday."集中提炼了核心消息:中国批准三种中药产品上市用以治疗新冠肺炎,交代了谁何时于何地做了什么、怎样做、为什么,各大新闻要素俱全。再次,主体部分续以另外三个自然小段,分别介绍特殊审批程序、药品类型来源和一线实践的检验、三种中药的专业名称,按照西方读者的关注程度和阅读兴趣,各小段新闻事实的重要性逐渐减弱。

2. 体现样式

新闻的本质是一种信息文本,它的主要功能是向读者传递准确的信息,因此新闻语言首先必须准确、客观、简明、务实。同时,为了有效传递信息,新闻需要吸引读者的注意,其语言也要具备通俗、易懂、具体、生动的特点。基于上述特点,新闻语言具有特殊的体现样式。下面,我们从时间表述、引语使用、多同位语和插入语的长句使用三个方面进行汉英新闻语言的对比分析。

1）时间表述

"Yesterday's newspaper is only good for wrapping fish."这是报界流行的一句话。从中可看出，新闻贵在新，时新性是新闻价值的重要因素。因此，记者们都会抢发当日新闻。据相关统计，英语新闻几乎全部使用了"today"或者具体星期几，而汉语新闻除了使用具体日期或周几，也常使用"近日""日前""最近""不久前""新近"等模糊用语，存在不交代时间因素的情况。

[例1] 日前，国家药品监督管理局通过特别审批程序应急批准中国中医科学院中医临床基础医学研究所的清肺排毒颗粒、广东一方制药有限公司的化湿败毒颗粒、山东步长制药股份有限公司的宣肺败毒颗粒上市。

对比句：China has approved three traditional Chinese medicine (TCM) products for sale to help treat COVID-19, the government's National Medical Products Administration announced on Wednesday.

分析：如上例所示，第一篇平行语料的汉语新闻时间表述是"日前"，而英语新闻时间表述是"on Wednesday"，更为精确具体。

2）引语使用

引语是新闻的重要组成部分，通常可分为直接引语、间接引语和部分引语三种类型。引语是新闻人物重要的原话或对其原话的转述，大多来自记者的采访，或是新闻现场的记录，可以大大提高新闻的客观真实性，也能使新闻更加具体生动。汉英新闻语料中都出现了高频率引用，且英语新闻更倾向于使用直接引语，以第一篇平行语料为例，汉语新闻出现一次直接引语，而英语新闻则出现了四次。以下以第三篇汉语语料（《中国医疗队为喀麦隆贫困群众提供免费救治》）和对应的第三篇英语语料"Chinese Medical Team Provides Free Health Care Services in Rural Cameroon"为例说明多种不同引语的混合使用。

[例2] 来自附近村庄的63岁的理查德·梅科加（Richard Mekoga）称，他患有背痛、眼睛和神经问题。"这是我第一次参加（中国）健康运动。我对我们收到的方式非常满意，"梅科加说。该男子强调，他确信中国医疗队提供的药物能救他。

对比句：Among them was 63-year-old Richard Mekoga who came from a neighboring village. Mekoga said he was suffering from back pain and eye and nerve problems.

"This is my first time participating in the (Chinese) health campaign. I was extremely satisfied with how we were received, " Mekoga said, adding that he was certain the medicine provided by the Chinese medical team will save him.

　　分析： 这里首先使用的是间接引语，客观转述村民理查德·梅科加身患的一些疾病。然后记者又在引号中引述了梅科加的两句原话，通过第一人称生动地体现了他受到中国医疗队特别援助后既激动又满意的心情，这是直接引语。最后又通过追加转述该村民的部分引语，表明了他对中国医疗队医生和药物的坚定信心。

　　3）多同位语和插入语的长句使用

　　英语新闻中的句子结构紧凑，信息量大，带扩展成分的长句较多，语法结构也比较复杂，常常采用一些关系代词、关系副词、连词等引导从句和并列复合句，长句中尤其多见同位语和插入语的使用。我们以汉语第四篇语料《中医药防治新冠肺炎发挥了哪些作用？》和对应的英语语料为例说明。

　　[例3] 中医药局党组书记余艳红介绍，全国新冠肺炎确诊病例中有 74 187 人使用了中医药，占91.5%。从临床疗效观察来看，中医药总有效率达90%以上。

　　对比句：A total of 74, 187 confirmed patients, which account for 91. 5 percent of the total infections on the Chinese mainland, have been administered traditional Chinese medicine (TCM) as part of their treatment, and over 90 percent of them have shown improvement during clinical observation, according to Yu Yanhong, Party secretary and top official of the National Administration of Traditional Chinese Medicine.

　　分析： 英译为一句长句，结构紧凑，信息量大，其中"which"引导一个非限制性定语从句，作为插入语成分来修饰"A total of 74, 187 confirmed patients"。"Party secretary and top official of the National Administration of Traditional Chinese Medicine"则是前面"Yu Yanhong"的同位语，介绍了引语来源新闻人物的身份。

二、篇章译写的特点和策略

　　汉英新闻报道在篇章结构和体现样式上存在一定的差异性。为了讲好中医药故事，传播中国声音，还需注重内外有别，基于海外受众的思维特点、阅读方式、中医知识背景以及信息需求，英译前对汉语的中医药新闻进行增删、重组、编辑、加工等译前处理，对接国外惯用的话语体系和表达方式。下面以汉英平行新闻语料第二篇《中医药服务"一带一路"沿线人民健康》和"China Focus：TCM Gains Popularity Among Belt and Road Countries"为例，分别探讨重组、省译和增译三种翻译策略的应用。

　　1. 重组

　　汉语新闻习惯先介绍背景信息，从一般到具体，从宏观到微观。英语新闻习惯开门见山,段首使用主题句,关键信息点靠前,背景信息补充在后。

[例4] 作为2022年中国国际服务贸易交易会期间举办的论坛之一,第五届"一带一路"中医药发展论坛2日以线上线下结合的方式举行。中国国家中医药管理局局长于文明在致辞中说,中医药已传播至196个国家和地区,成为中国与东盟、欧盟、非盟以及上合组织、金砖国家等地区和组织合作的重要领域。

对比句:Yu Wenming, head of the National Administration of Traditional Chinese Medicine (NATCM), said on Friday that TCM has evolved into a significant international collaboration field and expanded to 196 countries and regions. Yu delivered his comments at the fifth Belt and Road Forum for TCM Development, a themed forum of the 2022 China International Fair for Trade in Services.

分析:汉语新闻首先介绍了第五届"一带一路"中医药发展论坛的性质、举办的日期和方式。接着引出中医药管理局局长于文明的重要讲话精神。与之不同的是,英译新闻直接以于文明开头,亮明身份,转述他在论坛上的重要讲话。第一句构成这一段新闻事实的主题句,然后才在第二个句子中以补充背景的方式,介绍了该论坛的相关信息,构成新闻事实的支持句。

2. 减译

对外英语新闻报道的受众读者以目的语国家的民众为主,新闻翻译中往往可以略去他们关注度不高或是过于专业的信息表述,这么做的同时也能增强新闻的通俗性和可读性,提高新闻信息传递接收的效率。

[例5] 中医药交流合作已成为共建"一带一路"高质量发展的新亮点。2022年1月发布的《推进中医药高质量融入共建"一带一路"发展规划(2021—2025年)》提出,"十四五"时期,中国将与共建"一带一路"国家合作建设30个高质量中医药海外中心。

对比句:During the 14th Five-Year Plan period (2021 – 2025), China aims to jointly establish 30 high-quality TCM centers with countries along the Belt and Road, according to a plan issued by central government agencies, including the NATCM, in January.

分析:汉语新闻中的《推进中医药高质量融入共建"一带一路"发展规划(2021—2025年)》在平行英语新闻中被简化为"a plan issued by central government agencies, including the NATCM",专业的规划名称被略去和模糊化,使用了通俗易懂的大众化语言"plan",降低了阅读难度,真正使受众听得懂、听得进。

3. 增译

语言是传播文化的载体,对外新闻报道是向世界展示和传播优秀中国文化的重要媒介。当新闻的读者变成外国人时,他们对于一些在中国家喻户晓的事情可能知之甚少,或者一无所知。因此,对于境外读者存在理解困难的新闻事实,有必要增加背景知识。

[例6]　在常规临床治疗外,刘清国和其他中医还会给外国患者介绍中医理念,带他们到中医中心开设的练功房练气功、打太极拳。

对比句：As more patients developed their interest in TCM culture, Liu and his colleagues showed them Qigong and Tai Chi in the center's practice room. These traditional Chinese martial arts focus on exploiting the human body's inner energy to achieve physical and mental harmony.

分析：汉语使用者对气功、太极拳从小耳熟能详,因此汉语新闻中无须对其深入解释。而英语新闻语篇中的对比句第二句"These traditional Chinese martial arts focus on exploiting the human body's inner energy to achieve physical and mental harmony."是新增的译文,旨在进一步解释中医文化负载词"Qigong"和"Tai Chi"的内涵和功效,帮助不同文化背景的新闻读者更好地了解中医药文化,了解中国文化。

在翻译实践中,通常需要综合运用以上几种策略。比如例 4 中有重组也有减译,例 5 中有减译也有重组,例 6 中有增译也有减译。

第三节　段落的翻译

在完成语篇层面的内容和结构调整后,还需进一步对比汉英新闻报道在段落层面上结构和内容上的差异,并按照英语新闻规范对每段内容和结构进行相应调整。这里分别从新闻标题、新闻导语、新闻事实段落三个方面进行分析。

一、新闻标题译写的特点和策略

标题是新闻的题眼,它通常能起到概括提炼新闻内容、评价新闻事实、美化版面形式和吸引读者注意的作用。通过分析语料发现,英语新闻标题对比汉语新闻标题,具有两大明显的特征：一是常用省略,二是多用一般现在时。

1. 省略

英文词长、占空间大,为节省版面,英语新闻标题在语法方面往往能省则省。系动词、助动词、连接词、冠词等不表示实义的虚词通常都会被省略。下面以新闻语料标题举例说明。

[例1] 三种治疗新冠肺炎的中药颗粒获批上市

对比句:China Approves Sale of Traditional Medicine Products to Treat COVID-19

分析:完整的形式是"approves the sale of . . .",这里省略了定冠词"the",句子表达更简明。

[例2] 结缘中医·上中医举办第二届"中医汉语桥"

对比句:Second "TCM Chinese Bridge" Program Opens in Shanghai

分析:这里中文新闻标题分两个部分,用分隔号分开,而英文标题直接省略了"结缘中医"这一部分,只是翻译出体现新闻核心内容的后半部分。同时,规范的英语语法是序数词"second"前面要加定冠词"the",但在新闻标题中省略了冠词,简洁明了。

2. 时态

为突出新闻的时新性和现场感,对于过去已经发生的事件,英语新闻标题中多采用一般现在时态来表达,而不是使用过去时态或完成时态。

[例3] 中医药服务"一带一路"沿线人民健康

对比句:China Focus: TCM Gains Popularity Among Belt and Road Countries

分析:此处英语新闻标题谓语动词没用使用过去时"gained"或完成时"has gained",而是使用了一般现在时"gains",具有更强的即时感,体现新闻事件的影响正在发生和延续。

[例4] 中国医疗队为喀麦隆贫困群众提供免费救治

对比句:Chinese Medical Team Provides Free Health Care Services in Rural Cameroon

分析:同样,为了体现新闻事实的时新性,这里英文标题谓语动词使用了一般现在时"provides",而没有对过去的、已经发生的事情使用过去时"provided"或完成时"has provided"。

二、新闻导语译写的特点和策略

导语是新闻的导读,通常出现在新闻的首段,提纲挈领,概括全篇。它以简洁凝练的文字表述新闻事件中最重要的内容,吸引读者的注意。在英语新闻导语译写中,要重点把握以下两个特点。

1．注重交代新闻来源

在导语部分明确新闻消息的来源和出处，可以提高新闻的客观性和可信度。英语新闻常用"say""add""announce""report""declare""according to"等引出消息的来源。中文导语一般将新闻来源的机构或讲话人放在句首；而在英文导语中，机构或讲话人出现的位置较为灵活，在句首、句尾或句中都可能出现。

2．语言朴实无华，浓缩精练

导语一般一句一段，简明扼要，用最经济的语言揭示新闻事件的基本要素。英语新闻导语较少出现生动的描写，少用副词和形容词，语言比较朴实，高度浓缩，十分精练。如美联社要求导语的字数尽可能控制在 25 词以内，最多不超过 35 词。下面从新闻语料中选取两则导语对比举例说明。

［例 5］　央广网北京 3 月 3 日消息（记者 宋雪）日前，国家药品监督管理局通过特别审批程序应急批准中国中医科学院中医临床基础医学研究所的清肺排毒颗粒、广东一方制药有限公司的化湿败毒颗粒、山东步长制药股份有限公司的宣肺败毒颗粒上市。

对比句：CNN—China has approved three traditional Chinese medicine（TCM）products for sale to help treat COVID-19, the government's National Medical Products Administration announced on Wednesday.

分析：这篇新闻的英文导语使用了"announced"这个说意动词，引出新闻来源，点明了发布消息的官方机构，突出新闻的客观性和权威性。中文导语中，"国家药品监督管理局"出现在句首，而在对应的英文导语中出现在句尾，跟在新闻的实质性内容之后。这句英文导语的用词和句式都很朴实简单，整个句子比较短，只有 23 个词。因为对于英语国家普通读者而言，具体的中药颗粒名称太过专业，在导语中未被提及，只是出现在后面的新闻正文中。

［例 6］　11 月 18 日，第二届"中医汉语桥"在上海中医药大学国际教育学院举办，动人的校园秋色迎来了一批新、老朋友。

对比句：Shanghai University of Traditional Chinese Medicine（TCM）held the second "TCM Chinese Bridge" Program on campus on Nov. 18, offering foreigners a fast track for Chinese language and medicine learning.

分析：这一则英文新闻导语由一个单一的句子构成，词汇基础，句式简单，句子较短，共用了 29 个词。新闻来源"Shanghai University of Traditional Chinese

Medicine"出现在了句首。中文导语中"动人的校园秋色迎来了一批新、老朋友"属于描写性语句,在英文导语中被省译,取而代之的是概括介绍汉语桥活动的举办意义,即"offering foreigners a fast track for Chinese language and medicine learning"。

三、新闻正文译写的特点和策略

紧接导语之后的是新闻的主体,主体部分通常是一段交代一个跟主题相关的新闻事实,重要程度呈倒金字塔式依次减弱。其中包含跟导语密切联系的各类型引语、围绕主题展开的支持性细节事实、必要的背景或解释、与该新闻有关的其他附加信息等等。每一段独立构成一个新闻事实段落,一个新闻事实段落常常仅有一个句子,多采用分段符在版面上进行明显分隔。汉语重意合,英语更重形合。在对新闻主体事实段落进行译写时,为达到逻辑关系明晰,需做好连贯和衔接。分析新闻语料发现,以下三种衔接手段较为常用,分别从第一、二、四篇英语语料中选取段落举例如下。

1. 主题词、代词衔接

[例7] The agency used a special approval procedure to green-light the three products, which "provide more options for COVID-19 treatment", it said in a statement.

The herbal products come in granular form and trace their origins to "ancient Chinese prescriptions", said the statement. They were developed from TCM remedies that had been used early in the pandemic, and that were "screened by many academics and experts on the front line".

The three products are "lung-clearing and detoxing granules" "dampness-resolving and detoxing granules" and "lung-diffusing and detoxing granules", said the statement.

分析:这里下划线标出的三个主题词都与新闻主题紧密相关,其中第一段中"the agency"指代前文中的"the government's National Medical Products Administration",与导语紧密衔接,引出药监局批准三种中药上市的新闻事实;第二段中"the herbal products"与第一段的"the three products"呼应衔接,补充中药的来源和实际应用等新闻事实;第三段直接以"the three products"开头,再次衔接,引出三种中药颗粒的专业名称这一新闻事实。全篇通过主题关键词实现了连贯的衔接。

2. 连接词衔接

[例8] As more patients developed their interest in TCM culture, Liu and his colleagues showed them Qigong and Tai Chi in the center's practice room. These traditional Chinese martial arts focus on exploiting the human body's inner energy to achieve physical and mental harmony.

In addition to routine therapy, the TCM center has also conducted academic exchanges with local hospitals and organized training programs for local doctors, according to Liu.

China has also teamed up with other Belt and Road countries on TCM to tackle illnesses, as shown by the exhibitors at CIFTIS.

分析：英语是注重形式连接的语言，连接词或连接短语是非常常见的一种连接方式，在新闻正文中也不例外。这里下划线标出的逻辑连接词"as""in addition to""also"分别引出三个新闻事实段落，体现了递进、并列的语义关系。

3. 引语衔接

[例 9] TCM has effectively relieved symptoms, cut the rate of patients developing into severe conditions, raised the recovery rate, reduced the mortality rate and boosted patients' recovery, Yu said.

XuanFeiBaiDu Granule can increase the lymphocyte recovery rate by 17 percent and the clinical cure rate by 22 percent in the controlled observation, according to Huang Luqi, an academician of the Chinese Academy of Engineering.

Liu Qingquan, head of the Beijing Hospital of Traditional Chinese Medicine, said that two TCM drugs—Jinhua Qinggan Granule and Lianhua Qingwen Capsule / Granule have proven to be effective in the treatment of mild COVID-19 cases, while Xuebijing Injection can help treat inflammation and coagulation dysfunction.

Zhang Boli, an academician of the Chinese Academy of Engineering, said that TCM treatment has significantly lowered the proportion of patients whose conditions turned from mild to severe. "None of the 564 patients at the TCM-oriented temporary hospital in Wuhan saw their health condition deteriorating into severe," said Zhang. "We have therefore applied TCM treatment to over 10,000 patients in other makeshift hospitals, and the rate of patients developing into severe conditions were substantially reduced," said Zhang.

分析：这篇新闻正文中连续四个小段都是间接、直接或部分引语，通过"said"和"according to"引用和转述四位与会权威专家的观点。这四个新闻事实段落通过不同类型的引语产生了自然流畅的连贯和衔接，起到了支持、强化、解释、扩展导语内容的作用，进一步揭示了新闻事件的意义。

第四节 词语的翻译

中医药新闻会经常出现具有中医文化和理论特色的中医药术语,为提高英语国家受众对术语的接受度,在对外新闻宣传中灵活采取直译、意译、音译、音译加解释等多种翻译策略。此外,英语新闻用词中会高频率出现说意动词,并经常使用简短生动和形象化表达的词语。以下从新闻平行语料中举例说明。

一、中医药术语翻译

［例1］ 清肺排毒颗粒、化湿败毒颗粒、宣肺败毒颗粒

译文:lung-clearing and detoxing granules, dampness-resolving and detoxing granules, lung-diffusing and detoxing granules

分析:这一组中医药术语出现在美国本土报纸上,术语的直译意思明确,清晰表达了这些中药的功效和品类,信息的可接受度较高,可读性较强。

［例2］ 气功、太极拳

译文:Qigong, Tai Chi (These traditional Chinese martial arts focus on exploiting the human body's inner energy to achieve physical and mental harmony.)

分析:气功和太极拳这两个体现中国文化的汉语词,可以说已经在全世界产生了相当的影响力。这类术语通常的译法就是直接用汉语拼音的音译。这里细心的记者考虑到存在一些不了解气功和太极拳的读者,增加了一句英文解释,丰富了中医药文化输出的内涵,提高了传播效果。

［例3］ 金花清感、连花清瘟

译文:Jinhua Qinggan Granule, Lianhua Qingwen Capsule/Granule

分析:这两个中药术语采用了音译加增译的翻译方法。中文药名直接使用拼音翻译,然后增补了颗粒或胶囊的药物形式,以使英文读者能大致明白它们是某种药品。这里没有对拼音部分表达的含义做进一步解释,目的是避免使新闻过于专业化而影响读者的阅读兴趣。如果受众不是普通大众,而是可能需要了解更多具体信息的行业人士,那么可以增加对术语的解释。以"连花清瘟"为例,可以借鉴海外版连花清瘟胶囊包装盒上的英文:Lianhua Qingwen Capsule (Traditionally-used Herbal

Product: Helps remove heat-toxin invasion of the lungs, including symptoms such as fever, aversion to cold, muscle soreness, stuffy and runny nose.）

二、说意动词

顾名思义,说意动词即可以表示"说"(say)的动词。前文中提到过英语新闻报道的一大语篇特征是包含大量各种形式的引语,这些引语需要丰富的说意动词进行直接或含蓄的援引和转述。不同的说意动词能传达不同的语气、态度、立场。因此,在中医药新闻译写中也要特别留意此类英文动词的微妙含义和修辞色彩,做到精准用词,正确传达新闻人物的立场和观点。同时,使用不同的说意动词,还能避免用词重复,增加文采,使新闻报道更为立体生动。

[例4]　国家药品监督管理局通过特别审批程序应急批准……

译文：China has approved ... the government's National Medical Products Administration announced on Wednesday.

分析：示例中汉语新闻没有出现明显的说意动词,平行的英语新闻则按照新闻常用表达惯例使用了"announced"一词,表示"宣布、宣称、通知"等较为官方的说意表达。

以下为常见新闻说意动词英汉对照(张健,2016:102)：

acknowledge（承认）

add（接着说,又说）

admit（承认）

affirm（肯定）

allege（宣称）

argue（争辩,主张）

assert（断言）

boast（夸口说）

caution（告诫说）

claim（声称）

complain（抱怨说）

concede（承认）

conclude（断定,下结论）

confess（供认,承认）

contend（争辩）

continue（接着说）

contradict（反驳,否定）

declare（声明,声称）

deny（否认）

disclose（透露）

elaborate（详细述说）

emphasize（强调说）

exclaim（大声说,呼喊）

explain（解释说）

go on（就是,接着说）

imply（暗示）

insist（坚持说,主张）

maintain（主张,认为）

note（谈及,表明）

object（提出异议,反对,反驳）

observe（评述）   reply（回答）

pledge（保证）   reveal（透露）

proclaim（宣告，声明）   state（声明，声称）

protest（抗议）   stress（着重说，强调）

reaffirm（重申）   suggest（建议）

refute（反驳）   tell（告诉，告知）

reiterate（重申）   urge（敦促，力劝）

remark（议论）   warn（警告说，告诫）

三、简短形象的用词

新闻英语的语言简洁明了、通俗易懂、生动具体。因此，它的用词也是简短、通俗、具体的，多用短小的简单词，少用较长的生僻词。与此同时，新闻写作者也常常借助形象化词汇来增加画面感，使读者身临其境，产生共鸣。这些形象化词汇通常都具有一定比喻性含义。

[例 5]   The herbal products <u>come</u> in granular form and <u>trace</u> their origins to "ancient Chinese prescriptions".

分析：这里"come"这个动词简单到不能再简单，十分通俗，可读性强。"trace"作名词表示"痕迹，踪迹，轨迹"，作动词表示"跟踪，追踪，追溯"，用词不长，却非常形象化，使语言生动活泼，栩栩如生。

[例 6]   通过特别审批程序<u>应急批准</u>……

对比句：used a special approval procedure to <u>green-light</u> the three products

分析：此处"green-light"用词简单却不枯燥。它作名词表示"绿灯"，作动词表示"开绿灯"，与汉语言的习语异曲同工，是一个非常形象化的暗喻，使新闻语言变得可爱，能增加生动性，提高读者的阅读兴趣。

第五节　翻译练习与任务

一、翻译练习

以下是中医药主题的汉语新闻节选，根据英语新闻报道规范进行必要的译前调整,并译成英语。

（1）

周一,教育部对网友的担忧回应称,这八所学校不在《世界医学院校名录》中并不会影响这些学校的毕业生获取医师资格。

教育部表示,中医药院校是中国高等医学院校不可或缺的重要组成部分,按照国家相关法律规定,中医药院校的毕业生有资格获得相应的学位,并参加执业医师资格考试。

这一事实,不会因为一个非政府组织管理的院校名录没有收录这些中医药院校而受到影响、发生改变。

（2）

澳大利亚和新西兰的研究人员发现,针灸可以极大地减少痛经的严重程度和持续时间。

这项由澳大利亚和新西兰研究人员主持的研究还发现,针灸也能缓解与痛经相关的头痛和恶心问题。

迈克·阿穆尔博士说:"我们的初步研究发现,在中国许多的研究中,经常使用人工针灸,而不是电流理疗来治疗痛经。这会减少对止痛药的需求,同时也会改善头痛和恶心等伴随症状。"

"改善伴随症状是我们之前没有预料到的,在未来我们将会通过更大型的实验进一步探索。"

阿穆尔博士是西悉尼大学国家辅助医学研究所的博士后研究员。

这只是一个涉及了74位年龄在18岁到45岁之间的女性的小型初步研究,结果发现超过一半的人接受针灸治疗后,痛经的程度至少减少了一半。她们接受了为期3个月的针灸治疗,但效果却持续了1年。

许多女性还表示,她们没那么需要止痛药来治疗痛经了,并且其他伴随症状也得到了改善。

根据国际杂志《公共科学图书馆·综合》发布的研究结果,伴随症状包括了头痛和恶心等。

痛经在医学界又被称为原发性痛经,常见于25岁以下的女性。它还是女性群体中最普遍的妇科问题。处于生育年龄段的女性当中,每5人就有4人会面临这个问题。

（3）

世界卫生组织在《国际疾病分类第十一次修订本（ICD-11）》中首次纳入起源于

古代中国的传统医学章节,该修订本将于 2022 年 1 月 1 日起实施。

中国工程院院士、天津中医药大学校长张伯礼说:"《国际疾病分类第十一次修订本(ICD-11)》的正式发布有助于我国建立与国际标准相衔接并体现我国中医药卫生服务信息的疾病统计网络。"

据国家中医药管理局消息,目前,我国与 40 余个外国政府、地区和组织签署了专门的中医药合作协议,在"一带一路"相关国家和地区建立了一批中医药海外中心,在 30 多个国家和地区开办了数百所中医药院校。

(4)

世界卫生组织日前发布的一份新报告指出,中医药能有效治疗新冠肺炎,对轻型和普通型病例尤其有效。

世卫组织鼓励会员国在其卫生保健系统和监管框架内考虑使用中医药治疗新冠肺炎的可能性。

世卫组织中医药救治新冠肺炎专家评估会于 2 月 28 日至 3 月 2 日以视频会议形式召开。

来自世卫组织 6 个地区办事处的 21 名国际专家围绕临床实践、科学研究和循证评价等方面展开研讨,对中方专家分享的 3 份报告进行了交流和评估,并于 3 月底形成专家评估会报告。

二、翻译任务

1. 下面是关于 2022 年 9 月 15 日"中医针灸与世界"主题展在伦敦开幕的一篇汉语新闻报道①和一篇英语新闻报道②,请进行对比分析,并思考、讨论新闻编译的译前处理策略以及翻译过程中在语篇、段落、句子及词语层面所做的翻译调整、采取的翻译策略及原因。

"中医针灸与世界"主题展览在伦敦开幕

2022 年 9 月 15 日,"中医针灸与世界"的主题展览在伦敦南岸大学卡克斯顿学府、伦敦中医孔子学院开幕。本次展览由伦敦南岸大学卡克斯顿学府主办,黑龙江中医药大学、世界针灸学会联合会、中国中医科学院基础理论研究所协办。展品包括图文、书籍和实物,内容涵盖了人类非物质文化遗产、中医针灸的历史、中医针灸的诊疗

---

① 来源:《欧洲时报》英国版。

② 来源:Chinadaily. com. cn。

技术、中医针灸传承与教育,以及针灸国际交流等五个方面。

伦敦南岸大学校长 David Phoenix 教授和副校长 Deborah Johnston 教授受邀出席了展览招待会。同时与会的还有淑兰中医学院汤淑兰院长、英国针灸学院王天俊院长、牛津大学中医药研究中心马玉玲主任等嘉宾。英国针灸学会、英国中医药学会、英国中医联盟等会员,以及社会民众等 50 余人出席了这次活动并欣赏了所有的展品。

伦敦中医孔子学院的英方院长许亦农教授主持了招待会。David Phoenix 教授在致辞中提到了中医和西医在理念上完全不同,在理论和诊疗上各有其特点,并对伦敦中医孔子学院在推动中西医文化交流方面做出的贡献表示高度赞赏与支持。Deborah Johnston 教授在致辞中重申了伦敦中医孔子学院的三个使命:促进跨文化理解与交流,帮助当地中小学开展正式课程中的汉语教学,在英国发展中医针灸和与其相关的替代医学。许亦农教授代表主办单位介绍了展览的宗旨和概况,并分别就各位发言者的讲话为起点提出了更多的看法。

近些年来,英国民众逐渐倍加关注健康、养生和非药物疗法,中医针灸也随之在英国受到越来越多的关注和认可。这次展览正是以此为契机向当地民众展示中医针灸的各方面内容。各位来宾纷纷表示,此次展览使他们更深入、更广泛地了解了中医针灸及其历史,对针灸的现状和发展也有了更深入的思考。展览将持续到 11 月 11 日,面向社会公众免费开放。

Exhibition "Chinese Acupuncture and the World"

The "Chinese Acupuncture and the World" exhibition was opened on 15 September 2022 in Caxton House / the Confucius Institute for Traditional Chinese Medicine (CITCM) at London South Bank University (LSBU).

With images, texts, books and acupuncture instruments on display, the exhibition covers five aspects of Chinese acupuncture—intangible cultural heritage of humanity, history of Chinese acupuncture and moxibustion, diagnostic and treatment techniques of Chinese acupuncture and moxibustion, inheritance and education of acupuncture and moxibustion, and international communications and interactions in acupuncture and moxibustion.

LSBU's Vice-Chancellor Professor David Phoenix and Deputy Vice-Chancellor Professor Deborah Johnston attended the reception. Also present were Director of the Shulan College of Chinese Medicine Professor Shulan Tang, Director of London

Academy of Chinese Acupuncture Professor Tianjun Wang, Director of Chinese Academy of Medical Sciences Oxford Institute Professor Yuling Ma, along with over 50 invited guests, including members of profession bodies such as the British Acupuncture Council, the Association of Traditional Chinese Medicine, and Chinese Acupuncture and Herbal Medicine Alliance UK.

Executive Director of CITCM Professor Yinong Xu hosted the reception. Professor Phoenix, acknowledging that Chinese medicine and Western medicine have their own distinctive features in theory and practice, expressed his great appreciation and support for CITCM's contribution to promoting communications and exchanges between Chinese and Western medicines. Professor Johnston reiterated the three missions of CITCM: to enhance cross-cultural understanding and engagement, to help local primary and secondary schools implement Chinese language learning and teaching in their formal curriculum, and to develop Chinese acupuncture and related alternative medicines in the UK.

Afterwards, CITCM's Co-Director Dr. Bo Sheng from Heilongjiang University of Chinese Medicine and the visiting scholar Dr. Bo Ouyang from the National Administration of Traditional Chinese Medicine respectively spoke to the audience, emphasizing that Caxton Acupuncture Clinic is a top acupuncture clinic in the UK, and expressing their strong willingness for future multi-lateral collaboration.

On behalf of the organizer, Professor Xu introduced the purpose and background of the exhibition and elaborated on what was mentioned by each of the speakers. He also expressed his sincere thanks to the Caxton House team for their industrious and professional work, and to all the guests for their participation in the event.

With healthcare, well-being and non-pharmacological therapies gaining popularity in the UK in recent years, Chinese acupuncture has also received increasing attention and recognition. This exhibition provides a chance to showcase Chinese acupuncture as an intangible cultural heritage of humanity. The guests at the reception commented that this exhibition enabled them to have a deeper and broader understanding of Chinese acupuncture and its history, and to reflect more on the current situation and development of acupuncture. The exhibition will remain open until 11 November to the public free of charge.

2. 从《中国日报》或《人民日报》海外版选择一篇中医药英文新闻报道进行编译策略分析,思考、讨论如何基于对外英语新闻报道规范传播中医药领域的重大事件、重大进展,更好地自塑中医药文化和中国国际形象。

三、扩展阅读

[1] 刘其中.汉英新闻编译[M].北京:清华大学出版社,2009.
[2] 张健.新闻英语文体与范文评析[M].上海:上海外语教育出版社,2016.

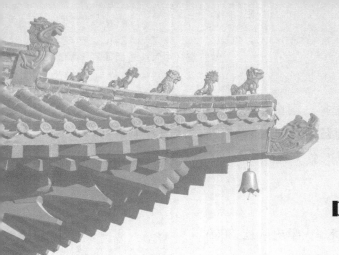

第四章
中医药科研论文译写

中医药科研论文（Research Articles，RAs）是中医药科学研究和描述性科研成果的载体。近年来我国中医药院校科研人员采取翻译或直接用英文写作的方法，不断将中医药科研成果以科研论文的形式推向国际并期待获得国际权威领域的认同。中医药科研论文属于专用科技文体，具有表述客观、逻辑严密、行文规范、用词正式、句式严谨的特点。为符合西方读者的知识背景和阅读习惯，实现科研论文的预期信息功能，我们可借鉴英文科研论文规范直接用英文进行论文写作，也可基于汉英科研论文文本特征对比进行译文调整。

第一节 语料导入

本章的中文科研论文语料来自国内中医核心期刊，英文语料选自 SCI 英文期刊论文。国内中医核心期刊论文能体现我国中医药科研论文水平，而 SCI 英文期刊论文反映了国际医学研究领域较高的英文学术写作水平，可以作为科研论文译写对比标准。入选语料库的期刊论文都要求遵循国际医学学术界规约，采取结构式形式。两篇用于语篇对比分析的论文分别是 CSCD 期刊《中国中西医结合杂志》中的《30 例湿热蕴结型结肠癌患者的肠道菌群结构变化研究》和 SCI 期刊《英国医学杂志》中的"Cardiovascular Safety of Non-Steroidal Anti-inflammatory Drugs：Network Meta-Analysis"。本节仅列出用于语篇分析的语料，段落和词语分析语料在第三节、第四节分别呈现，本节不再列出。

一、中文语料

·305·　　　　　　中国中西医结合杂志 2021 年 3 月第 41 卷第 3 期 CJITWM, March 2021, Vol. 41, No. 3

·临床论著·

30 例湿热蕴结型结肠癌患者的
肠道菌群结构变化研究

初　旭　脱璐尧　辛　红　徐　巍

摘要　目的　探讨湿热蕴结型结肠癌患者与健康人群的肠道菌群的差异。**方法**　30 例湿热蕴结型结肠癌患者的粪便样本做为观察组，收集 13 名健康人体检粪便样本为对照组，分别提取两组样本中细菌总 DNA，采用 16S rDNA 测序技术对各组的粪便样本进行分析。**结果**　与对照组比较，观察组肠道菌群中拟杆菌门、放线菌门、变形杆菌门、拟杆菌属、大肠杆菌/志贺氏菌属丰度明显增加（$P<0.01$）。Ⅱ期患者的双歧杆菌属、柯林斯菌属明显高于Ⅲ期患者（$P<0.05$）。**结论**　湿热蕴结型结肠癌与肠道菌群结构紊乱相关，关联度较高的为条件致病菌大肠杆菌相对丰度的升高，益生菌双歧杆菌相对丰度的减少。

关键词　16S rDNA 测序技术；结肠癌；湿热蕴结；中医证型；肠道菌群

Study on the Structural Changes of Intestinal Flora in 30 Colon Cancer Patients with Moisture and Heat Accumulation Syndrome　CHU Xu, TUO Lu-yao, XIN Hong, and XU Wei　*Department of Integrated Traditional Chinese and Western Medicine, First Affiliated Hospital, Harbin Medical University, Harbin (150001)*

ABSTRACT　Objective　To observe the difference of intestinal flora between colon cancer patients with moisture and heat accumulation syndrome（MHAS）and the healthy population. **Methods**　The fecal samples of 30 colon cancer patients with MHAS were selected as an observation group, and 13 samples from the healthy subjects were selected as the control group. The total bacterial DNA was extracted from the two groups and analyzed by 16S rDNA sequencing. **Results**　Compared with the control group, the abundance of *Bacteroidetes*, *Actinomycetes*, *Proteobacteria*, *Bacteroides*, *Escherichial Shigella* in the intestinal flora of the observation group increased significantly（$P<0.01$）. The contents of *Bifidobacterium* and *Collinsella* were significantly higher in stage Ⅱ patients than in stage Ⅲ patients（$P<0.05$）. **Conclusions**　Colon cancer patients with MHAS were associated with structural disorder of intestinal flora. Higher relativities existed in increased relative abundance of *Escherichiacoli* and decreased relative abundance of *Bifidobacterium*.

KEYWORDS　16S rDNA sequencing; colon cancer; moisture and heat accumulation syndrome; Chinese medicine syndrome; intestinal flora

结直肠癌（colorectal cancer，CRC）是常见的消化道恶性肿瘤，其发病率占所有恶性肿瘤的第三位，病死率居第二位[1,2]。诸多因素影响其发生发展和预后，其中肠道菌群结构和功能改变是重要因素[3,4]。中医药在结肠癌预防和治疗领域一直扮演重要角色，辨证论治是主要的治疗原则，其中湿热蕴结是其主要分型[5-7]，前期研究也发现结肠癌患者中湿热蕴结型占比较多[8,9]。肠道菌群是人体内种群数量最大和最复杂的共生微生物生态系统，被称为人类"第二基因组"[10,11]。肠道菌群失调可以直接影响宿主的肠道环境，诸多研究表明结肠癌的发生发展与肠道菌群的变化密切相关[12-14]。因此本研究以湿热蕴结型作为切入点，分析湿热蕴结型结肠癌患者与健康人肠道菌群差异分布的特点，旨在探讨中医证候与肠道菌群的相关性，寻找出结肠癌湿热蕴结型肠道菌群的特殊变化，为中医药预防和干预提供依据。

基金项目：黑龙江省中医药科研项目（No.ZHY2020-166）

作者单位：哈尔滨医科大学附属第一医院中西医结合科（哈尔滨 150001）

通讯作者：徐　巍，Tel：0451-85555815，E-mail：13796059990@163.com

DOI：10.7661/j.cjim.20210126.167

资料与方法

1　诊断标准

二、英文语料

BMJ

RESEARCH

Cardiovascular safety of non-steroidal anti-inflammatory drugs: network meta-analysis

Sven Trelle, senior research fellow,[1,2] Stephan Reichenbach, senior research fellow,[1,4] Simon Wandel, research fellow,[1] Pius Hildebrand, clinical reviewer,[3] Beatrice Tschannen, research fellow,[1] Peter M Villiger, head of department and professor of rheumatology,[4] Matthias Egger, head of department and professor of epidemiology and public health,[1] Peter Jüni, head of division and professor of clinical epidemiology[1,2]

[1]Institute of Social and Preventive Medicine, University of Bern, Switzerland

[2]CTU Bern, Inselspital, and University of Bern, Switzerland

[3]Swissmedic (Swiss Agency for Therapeutic Products), Bern

[4]Department of Rheumatology and Clinical Immunology/ Allergology, Inselspital, and University of Bern

Correspondence to: P Jüni, Institute of Social and Preventive Medicine, University of Bern, Finkenhubelweg 11, 3012 Bern, Switzerland juni@ispm.unibe.ch

Cite this as: BMJ 2011;342:c7086
doi:10.1136/bmj.c7086

ABSTRACT

Objective To analyse the available evidence on cardiovascular safety of non-steroidal anti-inflammatory drugs.

Design Network meta-analysis.

Data sources Bibliographic databases, conference proceedings, study registers, the Food and Drug Administration website, reference lists of relevant articles, and reports citing relevant articles through the Science Citation Index (last update July 2009). Manufacturers of celecoxib and lumiracoxib provided additional data.

Study selection All large scale randomised controlled trials comparing any non-steroidal anti-inflammatory drug with other non-steroidal anti-inflammatory drugs or placebo. Two investigators independently assessed eligibility.

Data extraction The primary outcome was myocardial infarction. Secondary outcomes included stroke, death from cardiovascular disease, and death from any cause. Two investigators independently extracted data.

Data synthesis 31 trials in 116 429 patients with more than 115 000 patient years of follow-up were included. Patients were allocated to naproxen, ibuprofen, diclofenac, celecoxib, etoricoxib, rofecoxib, lumiracoxib, or placebo. Compared with placebo, rofecoxib was associated with the highest risk of myocardial infarction (rate ratio 2.12, 95% credibility interval 1.26 to 3.56), followed by lumiracoxib (2.00, 0.71 to 6.21). Ibuprofen was associated with the highest risk of stroke (3.36, 1.00 to 11.6), followed by diclofenac (2.86, 1.09 to 8.36). Etoricoxib (4.07, 1.23 to 15.7) and diclofenac (3.98, 1.48 to 12.7) were associated with the highest risk of cardiovascular death.

Conclusions Although uncertainty remains, little evidence exists to suggest that any of the investigated drugs are safe in cardiovascular terms. Naproxen seemed least harmful. Cardiovascular risk needs to be taken into account when prescribing any non-steroidal anti-inflammatory drug.

INTRODUCTION

Non-steroidal anti-inflammatory drugs (NSAIDs) have been the cornerstone of pain management in patients with osteoarthritis and other painful conditions. In the United States an estimated 5% of all visits to a doctor are related to prescriptions of non-steroidal anti-inflammatory drugs and they are among the most commonly used drugs.[1,2] In 2004, rofecoxib, marketed as a cyclo-oxygenase-2 (COX 2) selective inhibitor, was withdrawn from the market after the results of a randomised placebo controlled trial[3] showed an increased risk of cardiovascular events associated with the drug. This finding was confirmed in other trials and a cumulative meta-analysis.[4] Since then debate has surrounded the cardiovascular safety of cyclo-oxygenase-2 selective inhibitors, followed by similar concerns about traditional non-steroidal anti-inflammatory drugs.[5] More recently, the US Food and Drug Administration decided against the approval of etoricoxib because of its inadequate risk-benefit profile.[6]

These debates and the patchwork of evidence resulting from multiple trials and cohort studies have unsettled practising clinicians.[7] Several standard meta-analyses were unable to resolve the debate because they failed to integrate all available randomised evidence in one analysis. Network meta-analysis allows a unified, coherent analysis of all randomised controlled trials that compare non-steroidal anti-inflammatory drugs head to head or with placebo while fully respecting randomisation.[8,9] We analysed the cardiovascular safety of non-steroidal anti-inflammatory drugs by integrating all available direct and indirect evidence in network meta-analyses.

METHODS

We considered large scale randomised controlled trials comparing any non-steroidal anti-inflammatory drug with other non-steroidal anti-inflammatory drugs, paracetamol (acetaminophen), or placebo for any medical condition. To be included, trials required at least two arms with at least 100 patient years of follow-up. In the case of trials with several arms, we included only arms with at least 100 patient years of follow-up. We excluded trials in patients with cancer. For an intervention to be included in our analyses, at least 10 patients allocated to

第二节　篇　章　的　翻　译

科研论文具有程式化特征,论文的体例和表达方式大致相同(方梦之、毛忠明,2018：81)。我们需要掌握汉英科研论文在篇章结构、语言特点等方面的差异,并在译写过程中加以注意,写出或译出符合西方科研论文规范的文章。

一、篇章的对比分析

1. 纲要式结构

医学研究科研论文一般遵循 IMRD(Introduction - Methods - Results - Discussion,即引言—方法—结果—讨论)结构,斯韦尔斯和费亚克(Swales & Feak,2012：285 - 286)对该篇章结构进行了详细描述(见表4-1)。

表4-1　科研论文 IMRD 篇章结构

结　构	主要内容和目的
引言	提供论文的理论基础,从对主题的一般讨论开始,逐步转向研究的特定问题、议题或假设。引言的另一个目的是引发读者对该话题的兴趣。
方法	以不同的详略程度描述研究的方法、材料/实验对象和程序。
结果	描述研究发现结果,并进行篇幅不等的评论。
讨论	以各种方式解释研究结果的意义,并提出一系列观点,其中部分观点能回答引言中提出的论断或问题。

科研论文每部分内容又可根据可识别的信息分为若干语步(move),有些语步是必须的,而有些语步不是。每个语步又可细分为次语步。因篇幅所限,本节仅以引言为例进行分析。引言部分的篇章结构称为 CARS(Creating a Research Space,即创造一个研究空间)模式(Swales,1990),每个语步的内容详见表4-2。

表 4 - 2   科研论文引言的语步构成

语步	目　的	手　段	是否必须
1	建立研究领域	表明该研究领域重要、核心、有趣或有争议	是
		介绍、回顾该领域以前的研究情况	否
2	确定待研究空间	指出该研究待填补的空白或待扩展的知识	是
3	占领研究空间	概述本研究的目的或研究性质	是
		列出待研究的问题或假设	否
		宣布主要研究结果	否
		说明本研究价值	否
		说明本论文结构	否

下面举例说明汉英科研论文的引言部分在纲要式结构上的差异。

[例1]   ① 结直肠癌(colorectal cancer, CRC)是常见的消化道恶性肿瘤,其发病率占所有恶性肿瘤的第三位,病死率居第二位。② 诸多因素影响其发生发展和预后,其中肠道菌群结构和功能改变是重要因素。③ 中医药在结肠癌预防和治疗领域一直扮演重要角色,辨证论治是主要的治疗原则,其中湿热蕴结是其主要分型,前期研究也发现结肠癌患者中湿热蕴结型占比较多。④ 肠道菌群是人体内种群数量最大和最复杂的共生微生物生态系统,被称为人类"第二基因组"。⑤ 肠道菌群失调可以直接影响宿主的肠道环境,诸多研究表明结肠癌的发生发展与肠道菌群的变化密切相关。⑥ 因此本研究以湿热蕴结型作为切入点,分析湿热蕴结型结肠癌患者与健康人肠道菌群差异分布的特点,旨在探讨中医证候与肠道菌群的相关性,寻找出结肠癌湿热蕴结型肠道菌群的特殊变化,为中医药预防和干预提供依据。(《30例湿热蕴结型结肠癌患者的肠道菌群结构变化研究》)

① Non-steroidal anti-inflammatory drugs (NSAIDs) have been the cornerstone of pain management in patients with osteoarthritis and other painful conditions. ② In the United States an estimated 5% of all visits to a doctor are related to prescriptions of non-steroidal anti-inflammatory drugs and they are among the most commonly used drugs. ③ In 2004, rofecoxib, marketed as a cyclo-oxygenase-2 (COX 2) selective inhibitor, was withdrawn from the market after the results of a randomised placebo controlled trial showed an increased risk of cardiovascular events associated with the drug. ④ This finding was confirmed in other trials and a cumulative meta-analysis. ⑤ Since then debate has surrounded the cardiovascular safety of cyclo-oxygenase-2 selective inhibitors, followed by similar concerns about traditional non-steroidal anti-inflammatory drugs. ⑥ More recently, the US Food and Drug Administration decided against the approval of etoricoxib because of its inadequate risk-benefit profile. ⑦ These debates and the patchwork of evidence resulting from multiple trials and cohort studies have unsettled practising clinicians. ⑧ Several standard meta-analyses were unable to resolve the debate because they failed to integrate all available randomised evidence in one analysis. ⑨ Network meta-analysis allows a unified, coherent analysis of all randomised controlled trials that compare non-steroidal anti-inflammatory drugs head to head or with placebo while fully respecting randomisation. ⑩ We analysed the cardiovascular safety of non-steroidal anti-inflammatory drugs by integrating all available direct and indirect evidence in network meta-analyses. (Introduction in the paper "Cardiovascular safety of non-steroidal anti-inflammatory drugs: Network meta-analysis")

　　分析：汉语科研论文引言较为简短，第①、②句阐明研究结肠癌患者的肠道菌群结构变化的意义，是第1个语步的第1个次语步，第2个次语步由第③、④、⑤句充当，概述该领域研究现状，即"发现结肠癌患者中湿热蕴结型占比较多""结肠癌的发生发展与肠道菌群的变化密切相关"。第⑥句表明本研究内容是"分析湿热蕴结型结肠癌患者与健康人肠道菌群差异分布的特点"，研究目的是"探讨中医证候与肠道菌群的相关性，寻找出结肠癌湿热蕴结型肠道菌群的特殊变化"。可见，中文引言缺失第2个语步，即没有说明以往相关研究的不足或有待扩展之处，导致读者无法充分了解开展这项研究的基础和必要性。相比较而言，英语科研论文引言较为完整地体现了CARS篇章结构，语步完整。第①、②句构成第1个语步的第1个次语步，说明非甾体抗炎药(NSAIDs)在管理骨关节炎和其他疼痛中的基石(cornerstone)作用。第③~⑦句为第2个次语步，按照时间顺序回顾非甾体抗炎药存在的问题和争议。第⑧、⑨句为引言部分的第2个语步，说明一些标准荟萃分析(standard meta-analysis)无法解决这一争论(unable to resolve the debate)，而网络荟萃分析(network meta-analysis)具有这方面优势，从而起到建构研究空间的作用。第⑩句概述本研究的研究内容是"analysed the cardiovascular safety of non-steroidal anti-inflammatory drugs"，研究方法是"by integrating all available direct and indirect evidence in network meta-analyses",为引言部分的第 3 个语步。

2. 体现样式

下面我们从常用句式、篇章正式度和人称三个方面对比分析汉英论文引言部分的体现样式。

1）常用句式

英语科研论文的语言表达较为固定,引言部分也如此(见表 4-3)。这些表达具有标识语步的交际功能,也可提升表达的地道性。中医药英文科研论文译写者需多加练习、熟练掌握。

表 4-3　英语科研论文常用语言表达

语步	交际功能	常 用 句 型
1	研究意义和必要性	... has been extensively studied.
		There has been growing interest in ...
		Recent studies have focused on ...
		... has become a major issue.
		... remains a serious problem.
		There has been increasing concern ...
		... has been investigated by many researchers.
		... has become an important aspect of ...
	以往研究回顾	... reported that ...
		These investigators demonstrated that ...
		A growing body of data shows that ...
		The findings supporting this conclusion come from ...
2	以往研究不足之处,建立待研究空间	However, little information / attention / work / data / research ...
		However, few studies / investigations / researchers / attempts ...
		No studies / data / calculations to date have ...
		None of these studies / findings / calculations have ...
		To the best of my knowledge ...

语步	交际功能	常　用　句　型
2	以往研究不足之处，建立待研究空间	Research has tended to focus on . . . , rather than on . . .
		These studies have emphasized . . . , as opposed to . . .
		Although considerable research has been devoted to . . . , rather less attention has been paid to . . .
3	交代本研究内容或目的	The aim of the present paper is to give . . .
		This paper reports on the results obtained . . .
		In this paper we give preliminary results for . . .
		The main purpose of the experiment reported here was to . . .
		This study was designed to evaluate . . .
		The present work extends the use of the last model . . .
		We now report the interaction between . . .
		The primary focus of this paper is on . . .
		The aim of this investigation was to test . . .
		Our primary objective in this paper is to provide . . .

2）篇章正式度

汉英科研论文的正式度都很高，英语科研论文的正式度体现在五个“多”：专业术语多、非言语符号多、名词化结构多、复杂长句多、被动语态多（王国凤，2014：180），如例 1 中的英语科研论文引言出现了“Non-steroidal anti-inflammatory drugs（NSAIDs）”“osteoarthritis”“rofecoxib”等专业术语；第③、⑨句等为复杂长句；第②、③、④句等使用了被动语态。同时我们也发现引言中不少句子是主动语态。近几十年来，科研论文出现了运用主动语态的趋势，主动语态具有表达清晰、明确、亲切的优势（方梦之、毛忠明，2018：79），值得中医药英文科研论文译写者关注。

3）人称运用

近几十年来，英语科研论文第一人称运用较为广泛，不仅用于评论较多的结论部分，在引言、方法和结果部分也较为常见（高芸，2018：78 - 83）。相比较而言，中文科研论文第一人称的使用频率较低。下面以例 1 中两个引言的结尾句为例进行对比说明。

[**例2**]　因此本研究以湿热蕴结型作为切入点,分析湿热蕴结型结肠癌患者与健康人肠道菌群差异分布的特点,旨在探讨中医证候与肠道菌群的相关性,寻找出结肠癌湿热蕴结型肠道菌群的特殊变化,为中医药预防和干预提供依据。

对比句:<u>We</u> analysed the cardiovascular safety of non-steroidal anti-inflammatory drugs by integrating all available direct and indirect evidence in network meta-analyses.

分析:以上结尾句都表明该研究的目的和研究方法。中文句用"本研究"作主语,客观性强;英文句用"we"作主语,将读者拉入协商过程。从与读者建立关联的角度来说,用第一人称复数有助于拉近与读者的距离,可能有助于构建学术胜任、值得信赖的学者身份,从而更好地为医学学术社团所认同。

二、篇章翻译的特点和策略

汉英科研论文引言的篇章结构和语言表达存在一定的差异,中医药科研论文译写者不能完全按照中文论文的结构和表达方式进行翻译或写作,还须借鉴英文论文写作规范,对汉语论文的篇章结构、语言表达、正式度和人称进行适度调整,以学术社团规约性的、读者易于接受的方式准确、适度地表达自己的观点,从而使学术观点得到国际同行认同。

[**例3**]　《30例湿热蕴结型结肠癌患者的肠道菌群结构变化研究》引言部分的英译

① Colorectal cancer (CRC), a common malignant tumor of digestive tract, ranks the third in incidence rate and the second in the mortality rate of all malignant tumors. ② Among many factors affecting the development and prognosis of the tumors, the change of intestinal flora structure and function is an important one. ③ Traditional Chinese medicine has been playing an important role in the prevention and treatment of colon cancer. Based on the main treatment principle of TCM syndrome differentiation, damp heat accumulation is the main type of CRC. Previous studies have also found that a large proportion of patients with colon cancer were diagnosed with damp heat accumulation. ④ Intestinal flora, known as human "second genome", is the largest and most complex symbiotic microbial ecosystem of human population. ⑤ The imbalance of intestinal flora can directly affect the host's intestinal environment. Many studies have shown that the occurrence and development of colon cancer are closely related to the changes of intestinal flora. ⑥ Therefore, in this study, <u>we</u> adopt the damp heat accumulation type of colon cancer as the starting point to analyze the characteristics of the differential distribution of intestinal flora between patients with damp-heat accumulation type colon cancer and healthy individuals. The purpose of this study is to explore the correlation between TCM syndromes and intestinal flora, and to find out the special changes of intestinal flora of this type of colon cancer, so as to provide the basis for TCM prevention and intervention.

分析：根据英文科研论文写作规范，第⑥句译文采用 we 作主语。为更好地符合规范，建议译写者在第⑤句的后面增加第 2 个语步，运用"however，..."等转折词交代以往相关研究的不足之处或需扩展的知识，然后引出待深化研究的内容或解决的问题。

第三节　段落的翻译

本部分以论文摘要为例，对比分析汉英摘要的连贯、衔接手段和信息流动方式，并基于差异进行译文调整。论文摘要是对全篇文章内容的高度浓缩和提炼，也是整个论文的精髓和灵魂（文师吾、谢日华，2012：10）。由于论文摘要是各国读者通过网络检索可获取的主要文献资源，不少非英语国家学术期刊都要求作者提供摘要英译，以获取更多受众群，扩大期刊国际影响力（王雪玉，2016：136）。科研论文摘要一般也遵循 IMRD 结构，保证译文整体的连贯性。下面我们从衔接和信息流动两个方面探究段落连贯性的实现方式。

一、段落的对比分析

1. 衔接与连贯

论文摘要和正文部分一样，具有正式度高、逻辑严密、层次分明、条理清晰的特点，需要经常表达逻辑思维的各种模式，例如时间与空间、列举与例证、原因与结果、强调与增补等等，因此英文科研论文摘要译写中，词汇衔接和逻辑连接词大量使用。

［例 1］　①肩周炎急性期，采用局部取穴、毫针针刺结合温针灸与主动功能锻炼，②慢性期局部取穴联合远端取穴、毫针针刺结合温针灸与主动功能锻炼为最佳

治疗方案。①

原译：① For periarthritis of shoulder at acute stage, the combined therapy of acupuncture at local acupoints, warm needling and positive functional exercise is adopted. ② At chronic stage, the combined therapy of acupuncture at local acupoints and distal acupoints, acupuncture with filiform needle and warm needling and positive functional exercise is the best program.

对比句：① As shown in the studies, the endotoxin-induced inflammatory response can be significantly inhibited by acupuncture whose efficacy can also be significantly improved by the manipulations. ② Collagenase pretreatment may be the first receptor to the mechanical force of the L&T manipulation. ②

分析：有些情况下，原文衔接关系是隐形的，语义却是连贯的，但译文中却需要选择使用一些衔接手段建立显性衔接，这种从无形到有形的转化在汉译英中尤为多见。汉语原文对比了肩周炎在急性期和慢性期不同的针灸治疗方法，但原译中没有用词汇显化这两种不同治疗方法。原译的另外一个问题是两句话的主语都比较长，导致句子头重脚轻，不符合英语句子表达习惯，也在一定程度上弱化了句子的信息效果。对比句主语"the endotoxin-induced inflammatory response"和"collagenase pretreatment"则分别清楚交代主要信息，连接词"also"也显化了句间逻辑关系。

[例2] ① 各组给予西药四联疗法；② B 组加中医辨证论治汤剂；③ C 组加抗幽合剂。③

原译：① All the patients received quadruple therapy; ② patients in group B took TCM decoction; ③ patients in group C took Kangyou Mixture.

分析：原文体现的是主旨—补充的关系，第②、③句可视为对第①句的补充说明。但是，原译没能准确把握原文的含义，误译为 B 组和 C 组只需服用中医辨证论治汤剂或抗幽合剂。此外，句子用分号表明的是并列关系，导致句间的逻辑关系不够准确。

---

① 选自：韩振翔,祁丽丽,褚立希,等.针灸结合主动功能锻炼分期治疗肩周炎方案的优选[J].中国针灸,2014,34(11)：1067－1072.

② 选自：Wang F, Cui G W, Kuai L, et al. Role of acupoint area collagen fibers in anti-inflammation of acupuncture lifting and thrusting manipulation[J]. *Evidence-Based Complementary and Alternative Medicine*, 2017(7)：1－8.

③ 选自：汪楠,王垂杰,李玉锋.中药联合"四联疗法"治疗 Hp 阳性慢性胃炎疗效观察[J].中国中西医结合杂志,2017,37(4)：406－409.

[例3]　方法：① 随机选取 153 例身体质量指数(BMI)>25 kg/m² 的多囊卵巢综合征(PCOS)患者,分为针灸组、针灸联合二甲双胍组、针刺安慰联合二甲双胍组,② 6 个月后比较 3 组治疗前后人体体征、临床血清学指标、糖脂代谢指标、排卵率及临床妊娠率。①

原译：Methods: ① One hundred and fifty-three patients with PCOS, whose body mass index (BMI) was more than 25 kg/m², were randomly divided into an acupuncture (A) group, an acupuncture plus metformin (A+M) group, an acupuncture placebo plus metformin (P+M) group. ② The changes in the physical signs, clinical serological marker, indexes of glucose and lipid metabolism, ovulation rate and pregnancy rate between the three groups were compared after six months' treatment.

对比句：① We did this phase 2, single-arm trial at 27 sites in France, Germany, Italy, and USA. ② Patients who had received two or more previous treatments received intravenous nivolumab every 2 weeks until progression or unacceptable toxic effects. ②

分析：实现科研论文的语篇连贯还意味着译者须基于对西方读者文化、思维和阅读方式的考虑,对原文的人称和语态进行适当调整。上例和对比句都选自摘要的方法部分,原译第①、②句都是被动句,显得缺乏和受众的关联,且头重脚轻的句子结构和冗长累赘的表达也不符合英语表达习惯。对比句由两个主动句构成,简洁明了,信息突出。

2. 信息流动和连贯

信息流动对提升篇章连贯性同样重要。篇章的描写一般由已知信息承担承上启下的作用,从而把篇章中所有句子粘连在一起,使篇章在意义上具有连贯性。因此,句子一般将前面提到的已知信息放于句首,作为讲述的出发点,也就是语法意义上的主语。信息型文本翻译一般采用信息聚焦原则,将信息由低值向高值排列,旧信息在前,新信息在后,举例说明如下：

[例4]　① 灸法具有良好的抗炎作用,② 灸温的高低直接影响治疗疗效,③ TRPV1 在感知灼痛温度(>43℃)后,参与了艾灸抗炎效应。③

———————————

① 选自：李荔,莫蕙,文斌,等.针灸联合二甲双胍治疗肥胖型多囊卵巢综合征不孕症的临床研究[J].中华中医药杂志,2014,29(7)：2115 − 2119.

② 选自：Rizvi N A, Mazières J, Planchard D, et al. Activity and safety of nivolumab, an anti-PD-1 immune checkpoint inhibitor, for patients with advanced, refractory squamous non-small-cell lung cancer (CheckMate 063)：a phase 2, single-arm trial[J]. *The Lancet Oncology*, 2015, 16(3)：257 − 265.

③ 选自：周攀,张建斌,王玲玲,等.不同灸温的艾灸抗炎效应及 TRPV1 作用机制研究[J].中国中医基础医学杂志,2015,21(9)：1143 − 1145.

原译：① Moxibustion has good anti-inflammatory effects. ② The temperature of high and low directly affects treatment efficacy. ③ TRPV1 in perception of hot temperature above 43℃ participates in the anti-inflammatory effect of moxibustion.

对比句：① EA can regulate hormone levels in the HPO axis and the spatial learning and memory ability in female SAMP8 mice. ② Moreover, this effect may have been more pronounced in the EA-Sanyinjiao group than the EA-Guanyuan group. ③ The underlying mechanism of the EA-induced changes may be related to gonadal hormone shifts in the HPO axis, followed by an improvement in spatial learning and memory. ①

分析：原译是对原文的逐句翻译，句子成分间关系松散，各句主语缺乏和上句的关联，信息流动和连贯性较差。对比句则信息流动流畅、逻辑清楚、表达简洁。第①句以 EA 为主语，新信息是 EA 的调节效果；第②句首先用"moreover"显化递进关系，句子主语"this effect"指代第①句中交代的 EA 调节效果，属于旧信息，并提出新信息，即调节效果在不同实验组中明显度不同；第③句从第①、②句提到的 EA 导致的变化出发，以变化的潜在机制为主语，说明变化产生的原因。

二、段落翻译的特点和策略

译者在译前应认真审视中文摘要的内容与结构，根据英文句群的衔接与连贯特征，做些必要的调整、删节或修改，避免出现句子重要信息不突出、缺乏逻辑性、条理不清等问题。以下是对上一小节选取的译文的改译。

[**例5**] ① 肩周炎急性期，采用局部取穴、毫针针刺结合温针灸与主动功能锻炼，② 慢性期局部取穴联合远端取穴、毫针针刺结合温针灸与主动功能锻炼为最佳治疗方案。

改译：① Shoulder periarthritis, at acute state, can be best treated by combining the therapy of acupuncture at local acupoints, warm needling and positive functional exercise, ② while, at chronic stage, by combining the acupuncture at local acupoints and distal acupoints, acupuncture with filiform needle and warm needling, together with positive functional exercise.

分析：改译将原第①、②句中的主语移到后面充当句子表语，恢复句子结构平

---

① 选自：Wang J, Cheng K, Qin Z et al. Effects of electroacupuncture at Guanyuan (CV4) or Sanyinjiao (SP6) on hypothalamus-pituitary-ovary axis and spatial learning and memory in female SAMP8 mice[J]. *Journal of Traditional Chinese Medicine*, 2017, 37(1): 96–100.

衡,并将两个句子主语统一为"shoulder periarthritis",将谓语动词合为"can be best treated by",第②句省略了主语和谓语以提升表达的简洁度。同时,用"while"连接前后句,突出肩周炎在急性期(at acute state)、慢性期(at chronic stage)不同的针灸治疗方法。

[例6] ① 各组给予西药四联疗法,② B组加中医辨证论治汤剂,③ C组加抗幽合剂。

改译:① All the groups received quadruple therapy, ②③ with group B and C taking TCM decoction and Kangyou Mixture respectively in addition.

分析:改译用"with"结构体现句子的主旨-补充关系,并增加"respectively"和"in addition"强调B组和C组分别要额外服用这些药。

[例7] 方法:① 随机选取153例身体质量指数(BMI)>25 kg/m² 的多囊卵巢综合征(PCOS)患者,分为针灸组、针灸联合二甲双胍组、针刺安慰联合二甲双胍组,② 6个月后比较3组治疗前后人体体征、临床血清学指标、糖脂代谢指标、排卵率及临床妊娠率。

改译:Methods: ① 153 PCOS patients with body mass index (BMI) above 25 kg/m² were randomly divided into an acupuncture (A) group, an acupuncture plus metformin (A + M) group, an acupuncture placebo plus metformin (P + M) group. ② After six months' treatment, we compared their changes in the physical signs, clinical serological marker, indexes of glucose and lipid metabolism, ovulation rate and pregnancy rate between the three groups.

分析:改译简化第①句中冗长的主语部分,用"with"短语替代"whose"从句,并在不影响论文研究客观性的前提下,在第②句中改用第一人称复数和主动语态,使整个句子显得简明生动、具有亲和力。

[例8] ① 灸法具有良好的抗炎作用,② 灸温的高低直接影响治疗疗效,③ TRPV1在感知灼痛温度(>43℃)后,参与了艾灸抗炎效应。

改译:① Moxibustion has good anti-inflammatory effects ② and its treatment efficacy is directly affected by temperature. ③ At a perceived temperature of above 43℃, TRPV1 participates in this effect.

分析:对原译进行改译时,在厘清句子关系的基础上,用"and"连接原文第①、②句,其中前半句主语"moxibustion"引出研究对象,宾语"good anti-inflammatory effects"为新信息,后半句用已知信息"treatment efficacy"为主语,引出新信息"directly affected by temperature"。第③句以上文提到的"temperature"为起点,通过将介词短语提前的方式,明晰新信息。此外,改译运用"its""this"等词汇衔接手段,加强信息流畅度、语义连贯性和结构紧凑性。

第四节 词语的翻译

目标受众接受度是译写者在用英文表达或翻译汉语词汇时考虑的一个重要因素。中医用语简明扼要,用字少而表意深,但如果翻译不当,对生活在不同历史、文化语境的西方受众而言很难引起共鸣。受众接受度还意味着科研论文译写者在表达个人观点时应力图表达谨慎,避免绝对化,防止引起读者质疑或否定。此外,译者根据词汇信息、逻辑信息进行语用推理的翻译策略能力也很重要。

一、中医药术语翻译

中医药翻译有特定的一套较为精确而又含义固定的名词和术语,这些词汇主要使用在病机、病因、诊断、治疗、方剂、针灸等方面(郑玲,2013:47)。译者在翻译中医药术语时,应尽量采用经典译法或当前通行的译法,以确保译文的准确性、严谨性和可读性。为最大化地传递原文信息,提升译文的可读性,译者经常综合运用直译、音译等异化翻译策略和意译、释译等归化翻译策略。

[例1] "三因制宜"实质探析[①]

译文:(Analysis on) Essence of Treatment According to "Three Factors": Climate, Locality and Individual

分析:论文标题有时会出现中医药术语,由于国外读者对很多中医药概念并不熟悉,所以为了使英文题目易于被对方理解,在译写英文题目时可以适当增加副标题,以便对某些题目中的名词术语进行简单的解释。

[例2] 目的:探讨中医通里攻下法对多器官功能不全综合征(MODS)时肠道屏障功能的保护作用。[②]

---

① 选自:郑玲.中医英语译写教程[M]北京:中国古籍出版社,2013:271.

② 选自:陈海龙,吴咸中,关凤林,等.中医通里攻下法对多器官功能不全综合征时肠道屏障功能保护作用的实验研究[J].中国中西医结合杂志,2000,20(2):120-122.

原译：Objective: To explore the protective effects of <u>Tongli Gongxia（TLGX）herbs</u> on gut barrier with multiple organ dysfunction syndrome（MODS）.

对比句：*Polygoni Multiflori* Radix is <u>the dried root</u> of *Polygonum multiflorum* Thunb officially recorded in the Chinese Pharmacopoeia as *HeShouWu*（HSW）in Chinese pinyin. ①

改译：Objective: To explore the protective effects of Tongli Gongxia（TLGX）decoction, <u>a traditional Chinese medicine for dredging interior and purging downwards,</u> on gut barrier in patients with multiple organ dysfunction syndrome（MODS）.

分析：原译采用的拼音加剂型名的翻译方法虽然比较简明，但是不懂中医的西方受众会一头雾水，字面之下蕴含的宣传和兴趣诱导更无从谈起。对比句首先对出现的拉丁语中药名"*Polygoni Multiflori* Radix"作了深化解释，使关于中医药的文化信息有了清晰交代，也使中国特色的拼音缩写表达在上下文中自然得体，更加顺应西方受众。改译也采取了深化翻译的方法，增加同位语，交代通里攻下法的功效。

二、表达可信度

汉英的修辞习惯不同，英语表达比较谨慎，而汉语喜欢渲染夸张。为避免引起西方读者的质疑或否定，科研论文译作者在表达个人观点时须留有余地，避免绝对化。

［例3］ ① 熟地黄粗多糖组<u>可显著</u>对抗造模所致动物胸腺和脾脏的萎缩，② <u>显著</u>增加模型动物胸腺皮质厚度和皮质细胞数，③ <u>显著</u>增加脾小结大小和皮质细胞数。②

原译：① GPRRP <u>can obviously</u> resist the atrophy of thymus and spleen induced by the model establishing, ② <u>can obviously</u> increase the depth of thymus cortex and the number of cortex cells, ③ can enlarge the size of spleen nodules and <u>obviously</u> increase the number of lymphocyte.

对比句：① Our data has further <u>suggested</u> that liver damage resulting from HSW-Ex consumption is dosage dependent in rats. ② It is <u>possible</u> that disruption in amino acid

① 选自：Xia X H, Yuan Y Y, Liu M. The assessment of the chronic hepatotoxicity induced by *Polygoni Multiflori* Radix in rats: A pilot study by using untargeted metabolomics method［J］. *Journal of Ethnopharmacology*, 2017, 203: 182–190.

② 选自：苗明三，孙艳红，史晶晶，等.熟地黄粗多糖对血虚模型小鼠胸腺和脾脏组织形态的影响［J］.中华中医药杂志，2007，22（5）：318–320.

and energy metabolism <u>might</u> lead to subsequent oxidative damage in the liver of rats.①

改译： ① The study <u>suggested</u> that GPRRP <u>could</u> obviously resist the atrophy of thymus and spleen induced by the model establishing，② increase the depth of thymus cortex and the number of cortex cells，③ and enlarge the size of spleen nodules and obviously increase the number of lymphocyte.

分析： 西方受众十分看重话语可信度。不管事实本身价值如何，有可靠、权威的证源和节制、冷静和含蓄的表述总是听起来更有说服力。最强烈的说法往往被人们拒绝，而最低限度的说法容易被接受。摘要原文①、②、③句用三个"显著"强调实验结果，并直译为三个"obviously"，这样过于肯定、强调的表达可能会引起受众不适。对比句第①句运用"suggest"，第②句运用"possible"和"might"，多样化地表达了作者态度的委婉和节制。改译后第①句增加"suggest"一词，委婉地陈述自己的看法和建议，并在"obviously"前加上"could"，做了必要的淡化处理。

三、根据上下文语境推理

信息型文本未知信息可以从语篇中已经发生过的事件中寻求线索、得出理解，因此，信息型文本翻译教学需要培养学生根据上下文语境对语义进行固着的能力，同时培养根据词汇信息、逻辑信息进行语用推理的能力，示例如下：

［例4］ ① 高血压病的<u>中医证类分布</u>痰瘀互结 900 例，占 59.68%；阴阳失调 544 例，占 36.07%；瘀血阻络 228 例，占 15.12%；气阴亏虚 184 例，占 12.20%；肾阳亏虚 131 例，占 8.69%。② 高血压病的<u>中医证素分布</u>血瘀 76.13%，痰 71.09%，阴虚 69.30%，阳虚 54.64%，气虚 37.93%，内火 7.56%。②

原译： ① <u>Syndrome</u> of intermingled phlegm and blood stasis is 900 cases, 59.68%; Imbalance of yin and yang is 544 cases, 36.07%; Blood stasis blocking collaterals is 228 cases, 15.12%; Deficiency of qi and yin is 184 cases, 12.20%; Deficiency of kidney yang is 131 cases, 8.69%. ② <u>Hypertension TCM syndrome factor distribution</u>: blood

---

① 选自：Xia X H, Yuan Y Y, Liu M. The assessment of the chronic hepatotoxicity induced by *Polygoni Multiflori* Radix in rats: A pilot study by using untargeted metabolomics method[J]. *Journal of Ethnopharmacology*, 2017, 203: 182－190.

② 选自：王丽颖,李元,李娜,等.1 508 例高血压病中医证候分布临床流行病学调查研究[C]//中华中医药学会心病分会. 中华中医药学会心病分会第十二次学术年会论文集,2010：192－198.

stasis is 76. 13%, phlegm is 71. 09%, deficiency of yin is 69. 30%, deficiency of yang is 54. 64%, deficiency of qi is 37. 93%, heat is 7. 56%.

改译：① <u>As for TCM syndrome distribution of hypertension</u>, there are 900 cases (59. 68%) of intermingled phlegm and blood stasis, 544 cases (36. 07%) of the imbalance between yin and yang, 228 cases (15. 12%) of blood stasis blocking collaterals, 184 cases (12. 20%) of deficiency in both qi and yin, and 131 cases (8. 69%) of deficiency of kidney yang. ② <u>The factors leading to TCM syndrome of hypertension include</u> blood stasis (76. 13%), phlegm (71. 09%), deficiency of yin (69. 30%), deficiency of yang (54. 64%), deficiency of qi (37. 93%), and heat (7. 56%).

分析：原译文在语法、标点符号等方面都有问题，其中第①句将"高血压病的中医证类分布"译为" syndrome"，第 ② 句将"高血压病的中医证素分布"译为"hypertension TCM syndrome factor distribution"，在语义和语法上都欠妥。改译时，通过利用句中提供的"中医证类分布"和"中医证素分布"例子准确理解术语的含义，并根据句中结构和上下文语境对术语翻译进行了灵活处理，分别译为"as for TCM syndrome distribution of hypertension"和"the factors leading to TCM syndrome of hypertension"。

第五节　翻译练习与任务

一、翻译练习

1. 以下表格①比较了世界中医药学会联合会的《中医基本名词术语中英对照国际标准》(*International Standard Chinese-English Basic Nomenclature of Chinese Medicine, ISNTCM*) 与世界卫生组织的《西太平洋地区传统医学名词术语国际标准》(*WHO International Standard Terminologies on Traditional Medicine in the Western Pacific Region, ISTTM*) 的脏腑术语英译，以及不同英译在《中医杂志（英文版）》(*Journal of Traditional Chinese Medicine，JTCM*) 与《美洲中国医学杂志》(*The*

---

① 来源：张喆,徐丽,闵玲,等. 基于语料库中医脏腑术语英译标准比较[J]. 中国中西医结合杂志,2023,43(1)：117 - 121.

American Journal of Chinese Medicine，*AJCM*）两本 SCI 期刊论文中的出现频数，请分析、讨论统计结果。

序号	脏腑术语	ISNTCM 英译	频数（总）AJCM 频数频次分布[次（%）]	频数（总）JTCM 频数频次分布[次（%）]	ISTTM 英译	频数（总）AJCM 频数频次分布[次（%）]	频数（总）JTCM 频数频次分布[次（%）]
1	脏腑	zang-fu organs	90 5（8.8）	85（58.6）	viscera and bowels	10 0（0）	10（6.9）
		zangfu organs	47 *0*（0）	*47*（29.9）			
		zang fu organs	13 *13*（22.8）	*0*（0）			
2	脏	zang-organ	13 0（0）	13（9）	viscus	1 1（1.8）	0（0）
		zang organ	32 *3*（5.2）	*29*（20）	viscera	59 19（33.3）	40（27.6）
3	腑	fu-organ	5 2（3.5）	3（2.1）	bowel	26 2（3.5）	24（16.6）
		fu organ	34 *20*（35.1）	*14*（9.7）			
4	五脏	five zang-organs	7 0（0）	7（4.8）	five viscera	15 5（8.8）	10（6.9）
		five zang organs	19 *2*（3.5）	*17*（11.7）			
5	六腑	six fu-organs	0 0（0）	0（0）	six bowels	1 0（0）	1（0.7）
		six fu organs	10 *2*（3.5）	*8*（5.5）			
6	三焦	triple energizer	19 2（3.5）	17（11.7）	triple energizers	0 0（0）	0（0）
7	奇恒之腑	extraordinary fu-organ	2 2（3.5）	0（0）	extraordinary organs	1 1（1.8）	0（0）
		extraordinary fu organ	0 *0*（0）	*0*（0）			

2. 指出下列摘要原译中的不当之处并修改。

（1）益气温阳、活血利水法对心衰患者神经内分泌的调节作用与血管紧张素转换酶抑制剂部分相似，有可能改善心衰患者的心室重构；通过抑制血小板的活性，可能对防止血栓的形成及改善心衰的进程有利。

YWHL showed a regulatory effect of neuroendicrine system partially similar to that of angiotensin-converting enzyme inhibitor, it possibly can improve the ventricular remodeling and would be beneficial to prevent the thrombus formation and improve heart failure by means of inhibiting platelet activity.

（2）目的：探讨麝香保心丸对心肌梗塞大鼠冠状动脉侧枝血管生成的影响及其机制。

The stimulate angiogenes effect and mechanism of Shexiangbaoxin Pills on coronary collateral development in the hearts of experimental myocardial infarction rats were studied.

（3）治疗原则为健脾益气、养阴生津、除湿降脂。

Treatment principles that strengthening spleen and nourishing qi, nourishing yin and generating body fluid and dehumidification and drop lipid were followed.

（4）24 只大鼠随机分成麝香保心丸组（A 组）、贝复剂与肝素组（B 组）和生理盐水对照组（C 组）。

24 myocardial infarction rats were randomly divided into 3 groups, 8 rats in group A were treated with Shexiangbaoxin Pills, 8 rats in group B were treated with Beifuji and heparin, and 8 rats in group C were treated with 0.9% normal saline as control.

（5）在发病因素与疗效的关系中，情志异常引起者疗效最好，总有效率达79.36%；更年期引起者疗效稍差，总有效率达 45.45%。

The disease caused by the disorder of emotion obtained the best therapeutic effect, and the total effective rate was 79.36%. The disease caused by the climacteric obtained the worst therapeutic effect, and the total effective rate was 45.45%.

（6）温针灸联合耳针埋压及单纯温针灸对肥胖并发高脂血症患者异常的脂质代谢均有良性调整作用，且温针灸联合耳针疗法在减肥作用和改善 TCC 和 HDL-C 水平方面优于单纯温针灸疗法。

Warm acupuncture combined with auricular acupuncture and simple warm acupuncture can both benignly adjust abnormal lipid metabolism of obesity patients with hyper lipidemia, and warm acupuncture combined with auricular acupuncture are superior to simple warm acupuncture treatment on antiobesity action and improving the TCC and HDL-C levels.

二、翻译任务

以小组的形式,从中医药重点期刊中选择一篇适合在 SCI 期刊发表的中文科研论文、综述或临床报告,并译成英文。要求根据英文科研论文规范,对译文的结构、内容和语言表达进行必要的调整,并讨论科研论文写作应遵守的学术诚信和伦理道德。

三、扩展阅读

［1］Swales, J. & Feak, C. *Academic Writing for Graduate Students: Essential Tasks and Skills*［M］. Ann Arbor: University of Michigan Press, 2012.

［2］郑玲. 中医英语译写教程［M］. 北京：中医古籍出版社,2013.

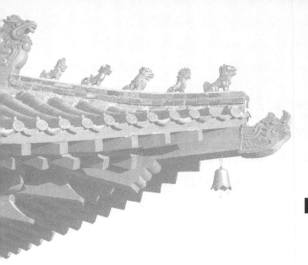

第五章
中医药科普读物英译

中医药英文科普读物是海外大众了解中医药文化的重要窗口。科普读物属于普通科技文体,具有科学性、通俗性和文学性的特点,语篇正式度比专用科技文体低,用词平易,句式简单,多用修辞格(王国凤,2014:189-191)。为促进海外受众的认知和理解,达到良好的传播效果,科普读物译者须注重海外受众的信息需求和文化背景,借鉴西方英文科普读物的篇章和语言特征,在传递中医药文化内涵的前提下,运用目标受众熟悉的话语方式和表达方式适当进行变通翻译。

第一节 语料导入

本章选取的中文语料来自《奇妙中医药:家庭保健顾问》《中国文化读本》以及"画说中医药文化丛书"中的《中医史画》和《药膳趣画》等国内具有代表性的科普读物读本。《奇妙中医药:家庭保健顾问》从百姓日常所需中医药知识入手,采取通信的形式,与读者娓娓谈心,具有很强的可读性(马有度,2009:序言)。该书曾荣获新中国成立60周年全国中医药科普著作一等奖。《中国文化读本》向国际社会展示了中国古代灿烂的文化和古代中国人的精神世界,写得明白通畅、富有情趣(叶朗、朱良志,2016:序言)。"画说中医药文化丛书"被列为上海市卫计委中医药发展办公室和世界中医药学会联合会推荐科普读物,以通俗易懂的语言、形象生动的绘画让更多人了解中医药文化,促进中医药走向世界。

英文语料包括 *Contemporary Introduction to Chinese Medicine—In Comparison with Western Medicine*(《打开中医之门：针对西方读者的中医导论》)、*The Web That Has No Weaver—Understanding Chinese Medicine*(《无人编织的网：理解中医》)，以及世界知名英文杂志 *Reader's Digest*(《读者文摘》)。《打开中医之门：针对西方读者的中医导论》从西方目标受众的角度出发，通过对中医和西医进行比较，运用通俗易懂的语言，全面、真实地向西方读者介绍了中医基础理论、诊断与治疗以及临床常见疾病。《无人编织的网：理解中医》是帮助读者了解西方和东方治疗实践的权威指南之一，语言通俗、深入浅出，为西方畅销科普读物。本节列出的语料主要用于语篇分析，没有列出的段落和词语分析语料将在第三节、第四节分别呈现。

一、中文语料(包括原译)

1.《治未病　大智慧》①

任智明先生：

① 来函敬悉，你读《周易》，有一句"君子思患而预防之"引起你的特别注意和思考。我很赞同你的看法，这个防患于未然的预防思想，确实很重要。对社会的"动乱之患"要事先预防，对人体的"疾病之患"也要未病先防。

② 对待疾病，首重预防，从源头上去治理，这就抓住了要害，抓住了根本。

③ 早在 2 000 多年前，我们的圣人先贤早已警钟长鸣：《黄帝内经》大声疾呼："圣人不治已病治未病，不治已乱治未乱，此之谓也。夫病已成而后药之，乱已成而后治之，譬犹渴而穿井，斗而铸锥，不亦晚乎？"

④ 说得多么好啊！疾病已经形成才去治疗，动乱已经形成才去治理，这就好像口渴了才去挖井，开战了才去制造武器，那不是太晚了么？！所以，只有在疾病形成之前就预先防止，那才是最好的办法。

⑤ 唐代药王孙思邈说得好："消未起之患，治未病之疾"，"常需安不忘危，预防诸病"。元代名医朱丹溪也强调说："与其救疗于有疾之后，不若摄养于无疾之先。"古代前贤为让广大民众牢牢记住"未病先防"，还采用诗歌来宣讲，邵康节的防病诗写得生动："爽口物多终作疾，快心事过必为殃。知君病后能服药，不若病前能自防。"现代的民间谚语也说得形象："洪水未到先垒埧，疾病没来先预防。"

---

① 选自：马有度. 奇妙中医药：家庭保健顾问[M]. 北京：人民卫生出版社，2009：6-8. 段落编号为便于分析添加，下同。

⑥ 圣人先贤"重预防、治未病"的指导思想,是维护健康最为重要的理念,面对当今的现实,面向人类的未来,都具有十分重要的战略意义。

⑦ 放眼当今世界,流行性感冒、病毒性肝炎这些流行病、传染病正在严重威胁我们的健康,脑中风、心肌梗死这些危险杀手正在夺取我们的性命。面对这两大类疾病的威胁,我们怎么办?根本的办法,就是加强预防,尽早预防,全民动员"治未病"。

⑧ 究竟怎样去预防?一方面,讲究卫生,改善环境,研制疫苗,加强群体预防;另一方面,又要讲究养生,保护精气神,扶正祛邪,注重个人预防。

⑨ 中医强调:"邪之所凑,其气必虚,正气存内,邪不可干。"讲究养生,正气强盛,即使流行病袭来,也可以减少发病;即使患病,病情也轻,康复也快。

⑩ 中医强调:"恬淡虚无,真气从之,精神内守,病安从来?"讲究养生,身心协调,许多慢性疾病也就难以发生。

⑪ 世界卫生组织的研究表明,只要实行科学、文明、健康的生活方式,做到"合理膳食、适量运动、戒烟限酒、心理平衡"这十六个字,高血压病可以减少 55%,脑中风可以减少 75%,糖尿病可以减少 1/2,癌症可以减少 1/3,寿命就能延长 10 年。

⑫ 看病难,看病贵,这是广大民众极为关注的热点。解决这个问题,固然要靠完善医疗改革,改善医疗服务,但要根本解决问题,还是要靠预防:"预防为先,预防第一"。人民政府"重预防",加大投入措施强;人民大众"治未病",注重养生保健康。在预防保健上投入 10 元钱,至少节省医药费 100 元,节省抢救费 1 000 元、10 000元……

⑬ 我们每个家庭,都应开设自己的健康银行,舍得健康投资,这是最为划算的投资。世界卫生组织与我国卫生部在北京联合发布全球报告的标题就是《预防慢性病——一项至关重要的投资》。更为重要的是,我们大家都要行动起来,人人懂得"重预防",个个都来"治未病",自己就能少痛苦,家庭就能多幸福,社会就能更和谐。在此奉上一首《养生防病智慧歌》:

> 看病难来看病贵,养生防病大智慧,大大节省医药费,
> 自己身心少受罪,家庭亲人少拖累,和和谐谐好社会。

⑭ 智明先生,"治未病"的战略思想,是前辈先贤聪明才智的生动体现,这智慧的光芒,穿过千年时空,至今仍然是我们应对疾病的指南。写到这儿,我不禁感叹起来:治未病,大智慧!

诚祝

安康　　　　　　　　　　　　　　　　　　　　　　　　　　马有度

2.《汪昂与〈汤头歌诀〉》①

① 随着方剂学的发展,专书越来越多,收集的医方也数量庞大,给初学者的理解和记忆带来很大困难。② 这时出现了一位医家汪昂,③ 他在其著作《汤头歌诀》中将复杂的中药药方,编成押韵的歌诀,非常适合吟诵和记忆。④ 如"四君子汤":"四君子汤中和义,参术茯苓甘草比。益以夏陈名六君,祛痰补气阳虚饵。除却半夏名异功,或加香砂胃寒使。"

⑤ 汪昂出生在明朝末年,早年爱好诗文,明朝灭亡后不愿为清廷效忠,才弃儒学医。⑥ 虽缺乏名师指导,但他凭借自己深厚的儒学功底,读了大量医书。⑦ 他发现很多著作都非常枯燥,不能让读者产生兴趣,所以他希望自己写的书,不但对专业学者有用,就连普通群众也能借此学习医药知识。⑧《汤头歌诀》一书收歌200余首,出版后果然深受欢迎,至今仍是医学启蒙的必读书之一。⑨ 汪昂也被后世看作一位重要的医学普及家。

Wang Ang and *Tang Tou Ge Jue*

① It's challenging for beginners to comprehend and memorize large numbers of medical formulas. ② A physician named Wang Ang versified formulas. ④ Take Si Jun Zi Tang (Four Gentlemen Decoction) for example, Wang Ang used six rhymed sentences to explain and supplement the formula, "There are four ingredients in this formula—Ren Shen (Radix et Rhizoma Ginseng), Bai Zhu (Rhizoma Atractylodis Macrocephalae), Fu Ling (Poria) and Gan Cao (Radix et Rhizoma Glycyrrhizae). This formula is called "gentlemen" because of their equal dose and neutral property. By adding Ban Xia (Rhizoma Pinelliae) and Chen Pi (Pericarpium Citri Reticulatae), this formula is called Liu Jun Zi Tang (Six Gentlemen Docoction), which acts to resolve phlegm, tonify qi and warm yang. By removing Ban Xia, this formula is called Yi Gong San (Special Achievement Powder). In addition, by adding Mu Xiang (Radix Aucklandiae) and Sha Ren (Fructus Amomi), this formula acts to circulate qi and warm the spleen and stomach."

⑤ Born in the later years of Ming Dynasty, Wang Ang loved poetry and literature. ⑥ After the fall of the Ming Dynasty, he started to learn medicine and read numerous

① 选自:"画说中医药文化"丛书编委会. 中医史画[M]. 北京:中国轻工业出版社,2018:124 - 125.

medical books. ⑦ However, he found these medical books very boring. He then decided to write his own books to attract more readers. ⑧ The Tang Tou Ge Jue (Versified Prescriptions) collected approximately 200 versified formulas.

3.《"生"的哲学》①

① 中国传统哲学是"生"的哲学。② 孔子说的"天",就是生育万物。③ 他以"生"作为天道、天命。④《易传》发挥孔子的思想,说:"生生之谓易。"又说:"天地之大德曰生。"⑤ 生,就是万物生长,就是创造生命。生生,就是生而又生,创造又创造。⑥《易传》的意思就是说,天地以"生"为道,以"生"为德。⑦ 后代的儒家思想家都继承孔子和《易传》的这个思想,强调人的仁心、善心,就来源于"天地生物之心"。⑧ 因此"生"就是"仁","生"就是善。⑨ 宋代周敦颐说:"天以阳生万物,以阴成万物。⑩ 生,仁也;成,义也。"⑪ 宋代程颐说:"生之性便是仁。"⑫ 宋代朱熹说:"仁是天地之生气。""仁是生底意思。"⑬ 所以儒家主张的"仁",不仅亲亲、爱人,而且从亲亲、爱人推广到爱天地万物。⑭ 因为人与天地万物一体,都属于一个大生命世界。⑮ 孟子说:"亲亲而仁民,仁民而爱物。"⑯ 宋代张载说:"民吾同胞,物吾与也。"(世界上的民众都是我的亲兄弟,天地间的万物都是我的同伴。)⑰ 宋代程颢说:"人与天地一物也。"⑱ 又说:"仁者以天地万物为一体。"⑲ "仁者浑然与万物同体。"⑳ 朱熹说:"天地万物本吾一体。"㉑ 这样的话很多。㉒ 这些话都是说,人与万物是同类,是平等的,所以人应该把爱推广到天地万物。

The Philosophy of "Life"②

① Traditional Chinese philosophy is a philosophy of "life." ② To Confucius, Heaven is the source of all living things. ③ He regards the "creation of life" as the "Heavenly Way" and the "Heavenly Destination." ④⑤⑥ *The Book of Changes* (*Yijing*), following Confucius' viewpoint, explains, "The continuous creation of life is change," and "The great virtue of Heaven and Earth is creating life." ⑮ Mencius (c. 372 – 289 BC), a great Confucian scholar who lived just over 100 years after Confucius, said, "(One should) love one's family, love the people, and love all living things in the world." ⑦ Confucian thinkers of later generations carried on the idea of "Heaven and Earth giving birth to all life," and thus emphasized love for and kindness toward all

---

① 选自: 叶朗,朱良志. 中国文化读本[M]. 北京: 外语教学与研究出版社,2016: 60 – 61.

② 选自: Ye L, Zhu L Z. *Insights into Chinese Culture*[M]. Beijing: Foreign Language Teaching and Research Press, 2008: 34 – 35.

living things. （增译） For example, many prominent Confucian scholars of the Song Dynasty (960－1279) echoed their master's view on life. ⑨ Zhou Dunyi (1017－1073) said, "Heaven creates life through *yang* and nurtures life through *yin*." ⑪ Cheng Yi (1033－1107) said, "The nature of life is live." ⑯ Zhang Zai (1020－1077) said, "All people in the world are my brothers and all beings in the world are my companions." ⑰ Cheng Hao (1032－1085) said, "Those with love regard themselves as the same as other living things in the world." ⑬ We can see from their thoughts that Confucian love starts from loving one's family and other people, to loving all living things in the world. ㉒ Humans and other living things are of the same kind and are equal with each other.

二、英文语料

1. Confucianism（《儒学》）①

Confucianism was initiated by Confucius (551－479 B. C.) who lived in late Zhou Dynasty or by the end of Spring and Autumn Period. He was a great thinker and educationist. The kernel of his thought consists of humaneness and the golden mean. His words and deeds were chiefly recorded in *Lun Yu* (*Analects of Confucius* or *Analects* for short). The book was compiled by his disciples after his death.

During the period from Pre-Qin time to the early years of Han Dynasty (from the 7th to the early 2nd century B. C.) various schools of thought emerged and competed for domination. In the 2nd century B. C. , the Emperor Wu of early Han Dynasty adopted Dong Zhongshu's suggestion to revere only Confucianism, but reject all other schools of thought. Since then Confucianism had been the major discipline of philosophy in the subsequent dynasties in China. It became the kernel of the feudal ethical code and exerted strong influence on the traditional Chinese culture.

1) Humaneness and Medical Ethics

A major part of the core of Confucianism is humaneness, which has given tremendous impact on Chinese medical ethics. Up till now, every Chinese doctor should always keep in mind that "medicine is the art of humaneness" since he or she began to

---

① 选自：Xie Z F, Xie F. *Contemporary Introduction to Chinese Medicine—In Comparison with Western Medicine*[M]. Beijing: Foreign Language Press, 2010: 3－6.

study medicine. Such highly inclusive and abstract statement has provided the fundamental guideline for ethics of Chinese medicine.

What is Confucian humaneness? The following citations from the book *Analects* will give the answer. "A humane person loves the people." "A humane person, in wishing to establish self, establishes others; in wishing to enlighten self, enlightens others. To be capable of appraising self in order to comprehend others can be regarded as the key to humaneness." "What you yourself do not want, do not distribute to others." "Do not impose upon others what you do not desire yourself."

A humane person loves people. This is an illustration to show that Confucian humaneness may be equated to Christian godliness. Here humaneness means "love the people" while, for the equivalent Christian slogans, "God is love, and he who abides in love abides in God, and God abides in him."

2) Opposition to Witchcraft

Confucius's negative attitude toward deity greatly facilitated the development of Chinese medicine by getting rid of magical and superstitious medical practices performed by wizards. In *Analects* the following passage was recorded: Ji Lu, one of Confucius's disciples, inquired how one should serve Spiritual Beings. Confucius answered, "We are as yet not capable of serving humans; how can we be able of serving Spirits?" The disciple went on, "May I inquire about death?" The master replied, "We do not as yet understand life; how can we understand death?" Chinese scholars usually maintain that justice and humaneness are the two pillars of Confucian ethics.

3) The Golden Mean and Methodology (Omitted)

4) Negative Impacts (Omitted)

2. Ancient But Still Alive(《古老而充满活力》)①

① Chinese medicine is more than 2,000 years old. Yet over all that time, it has retained an aesthetic and pragmatic relevance for humankind today. Of course, any tradition remains vital only insofar as it allows itself to grow and develop. The Chinese tradition is no different. Based on ancient and revered texts, it has continued to discover

---

① 选自：Kaptchuk T J. *The Web That Has No Weaver—Understanding Chinese Medicine*[M]. New York: McGraw-Hill, 2000: 24－26. 段落编号为便于分析添加。

itself anew.

② The *Huang-di Nei-jing* or *Inner Classic of the Yellow Emperor* (hereafter referred to as the *Nei Jing*) is the source of all Chinese medical theory, the Chinese equivalent of the Hippocratic corpus. Compiled by unknown authors between 300 and 100 B. C. E. , it is the oldest of the Chinese medical texts. The knowledge and theoretical formulations it contains are the basic medical ideas developed and elaborated by later thinkers.

③ The *Nei Jing* has been called the bible of Chinese medicine, and the rest of Chinese medicine can be compared to rabbinical exegesis interpretation of doctrine by church fathers. Just as, in the Jewish tradition, later authorities needed to explain theoretical issues raised by the Torah, so Chinese commentators added glosses on the *Nei Jing* that elucidated or even amended its seminal ideas. The Chinese medical tradition thus brings together folk remedies and the therapeutics of China's physician-literati who served the Imperial Court. It synthesized the medicine of one dynasty and another, one place and another, one thinker and another. Every dynasty has produced practitioners equal in stature to Galen, Avicenna, or Paracelsus, and all of them have made important additions and revisions to the tradition.

④ In China today, the primary textbooks used to train traditional doctors are contemporary interpretations and clarifications of Qing dynasty (1644 – 1911) commentaries. These books are, in turn, clarifications of Ming dynasty (1368 – 1644) reworkings, which are also reworkings of earlier material. This process goes all the way back to the Han dynasty (202 B. C. E. –220 C. E.). Such transmission through the dynastic pathway not only preserved and encapsulated the original sources, but also elucidated and reformed them.

⑤ It is for this reason that the *Nei Jing*, although it is the source of the tradition, is usually one of the last texts to be studied in contemporary schools of Chinese medicine. The *Nei Jing*, written in archaic language, is often unclear and inconsistent, and can only be understood after much preparation. Without the commentaries and modifications of later eras, the *Nei Jing* would be almost completely unintelligible. So the source requires the tradition to explain it, but both are necessary to guide Chinese theory and practice.

⑥ Within Chinese medicine, as in all traditional systems, there is a tension between that which is tacitly recognized as no longer useful and that which continues to be accepted as profound. <u>This book attempts to bring Chinese medicine to a Western</u> <u>audience, and because it does so within the ancient tradition, it is, finally, another</u> <u>commentary on the commentaries.</u>

3. Knocking Out Diabetes(《击败糖尿病》)①

Striking new studies show how you can control,

or even reverse, this common disease

When Michael Trailovici began feeling unusually hungry and thirsty, the 42-year-old editor didn't imagine they could be symptoms of a condition, let alone a serious one. He didn't see his doctor. That was in 1997. Today Michael, now 65, is one of approximately 416 million people around the world with type 2 diabetes.

Nearly half of those are unaware of their condition. The disease is so prevalent that the World Health Organization is calling it an "epidemic".

If type 2 diabetes is left untreated, or is not managed well, the consequences can be devastating. Risks include damage to the blood vessels, heart, liver, kidneys and eyes. It can also increase the risks of Alzheimer's disease, and lead to amputation—and even death.

According to Diabetes Australia, an estimated two million Australians are at high risk of developing type 2 diabetes.

But there is hope. Experts say that the numbers of type 2 diabetes cases are so high and climbing so fast due largely to our modern diet; this means the disease and its severity are mostly within our control.

Recent research has found that with attention to lifestyle and diet alone, these numbers can be reduced, and future cases prevented. In some cases, we may even be able to force the illness into remission. Here is the latest research on type 2 diabetes and diet. There are some actions you can take to help reduce your chances of developing it, and if you have already been diagnosed, how to maintain control.

WHAT IT'S ALL ABOUT

It starts with sugar. Cells throughout your body need it, in the form of glucose, as a fuel in order to function. But for the glucose to get past the cells' membranes, it needs a

---

① 选自：Bartholomew A. Knocking Out Diabetes[J]. *Reader's Digest Australia*, Dec. 2020: 42 – 49.

"key" to get in. Insulin is that key.

When a person has type 2 diabetes, their body produces enough insulin, at least at first—this is unlike type 1 diabetes, when the pancreas fails to produce much or any insulin. But in type 2 diabetes, though they produce insulin, their body is "resistant" to using it. The insulin key doesn't work. The cells have trouble recognising the insulin and resist the cell to open up.

When glucose can't get where it's needed, it keeps circulating in the blood, acting as an inflammatory agent, slowly but relentlessly causing damage.

HOW CAN I HAVE DIABETES? (Omitted)

DIET AND DIABETES (Omitted)

OVER 65s TAKE NOTE (Omitted)

DON'T LET DIABETES WIN (Omitted)

第二节 篇章的翻译

一、篇章的对比分析

1. 纲要式结构

通过汉英平行文本对比,我们可以了解汉英科普读物在语篇结构和语言特点上的主要差异。

1)《治未病 大智慧》与"Confucianism""Ancient But Still Alive"和"Knocking Out Diabetes"纲要式结构对比分析

分析:对比发现汉英文本的语篇结构各有特点。《治未病 大智慧》共计 14 段,每段较短且无明显的主题句。经分析后发现,全文围绕六个方面展开:作者在开头段寒暄和问候后,在第 2~5 段阐述圣人先贤"重预防、治未病"的指导思想,第 6~7 段说明"重预防、治未病"思想对当今现实和人类未来的重要意义,第 8~11 段提出具体的重预防、治未病措施,第 12~13 段指出该思想对于当前构建和谐社会的意义,第 14 段进行全文总结。可见,《治未病 大智慧》一文虽结构比较松散,但内容层层递进,主题思想明确。

"Confucianism"一文语篇结构清晰,段落主题明显。全文采取总分结构,总起段简要介绍了孔子的生活年代、主要主张等等,着重论述了儒家思想是中国封建伦理道德的核心,对中国传统文化具有深刻影响。正文部分由四个小节构成,并配有小标题"Humaneness and Medical Ethics""Opposition to Witchcraft""The Golden Mean and Methodology""Negative Impacts",分别说明人道主义与医学伦理、反对巫术、中庸之道以及负面作用四个方面的内容。"Ancient But Still Alive"一文论述了中医为什么古老而依旧充满生命力。全文共六个段落,每个段落主题明显(主题句如下划线所示),内容层层递进。首段开门见山,指出中医通过典籍保持生命力,第2段指明《黄帝内经》是中医理论的基础,第3段说明这部典籍经历了不同朝代的不断修订,第4段进而说明历朝历代所作的修订不仅保存了原著的思想,还不断阐明和改革,第5段指出典籍需要用中医传统进行解释,两者对于中医理论和实践都是必要的,第6段基于以上段落的阐述,指出本书也是基于传统对中医的再次阐述。

"Knocking Out Diabetes"的语篇结构清晰,段落主题明显,全文分为引言和正文两大部分,引言描述了全球糖尿病患者的现状和该病的严重性,最后两句"Here is the latest research on type 2 diabetes and diet. There are some actions you can take to help reduce your chances of developing it, and if you have already been diagnosed, how to maintain control."起到承上启下的作用。正文由五个小节构成,并配有小标题:"WHAT IT'S ALL ABOUT""HOW CAN I HAVE DIABETES?""DIET AND DIABETES""OVER 65s TAKE NOTE""DON'T LET DIABETES WIN",分别说明糖尿病的基本知识、患病原因、饮食和糖尿病的关系、65岁以上人群注意事项,最后提出战胜糖尿病的号召。分析可见,中文文本采取通信的形式,虽然形式比较松散,但内容连贯、语义流畅,而英文文本结构严密、逻辑清晰,采用小标题或主题句的形式凸显主题。

2)《汪昂与〈汤头歌诀〉》原文与原译纲要式结构分析

分析:《汪昂与〈汤头歌诀〉》第一段直接介绍汪昂将复杂的"四君子汤"药方编成押韵歌诀的例子,第二段介绍汪昂的经历、编写歌诀的原因、取得的成就及后世对他的评价。原译遵循和原文一样的语篇结构。英文读物一般遵循"general—specific"(笼统—具体)的篇章结构,即文章开头段提供背景知识、引入讨论话题、交代文章主题,然后正文段提供细节、进行解释说明,最后进行全文总结。

2. 体现样式

汉英科普读物平行文本都充分体现了科普读物语言的科学性、通俗性和文学性特点,下文从《治未病 大智慧》、"Knocking Out Diabetes"和"Confucianism"中举例说明如下。

[**例1**] 世界卫生组织的研究表明,只要实行科学、文明、健康的生活方式,做到"合理膳食、适量运动、戒烟限酒、心理平衡"这十六个字,高血压病可以减少 <u>55%</u>,脑中风可以减少 <u>75%</u>,糖尿病可以减少 <u>1/2</u>,癌症可以减少 <u>1/3</u>,寿命就能延长 <u>10 年</u>。

对比句: As well as hunger and thirst, <u>early symptoms can include fatigue, weight loss, frequent urination and blurry vision</u>.

分析:科学性是科普文体的第一特征。科普翻译作为普及科学知识、传播科学思想和弘扬科学精神的一个重要途径,其蕴含的科学知识应该是准确无误的,其文字逻辑应该是严密、经得起推敲的(王国凤,2014:189)。汉英平行文本列举的数字和糖尿病症状都体现了专业用语准确的特点,确保其蕴含的科学知识准确无误。

[**例2**] <u>说得多么好啊!</u>疾病已经形成才去治疗,动乱已经形成才去治理,这就<u>好像口渴了才去挖井,开战了才去制造武器,那不是太晚了么</u>?! 所以,只有在疾病形成之前就预先防止,那才是最好的办法。

对比句 1: <u>But what does meat have to do with blood sugar?</u> <u>Our</u> cells' membranes are comprised, in part, of fat, which comes from what <u>we</u> eat.

对比句 2: <u>What is Confucian humaneness?</u> The following citations from the book *Analects* will give the answer.

分析:为增强科普读物的可读性,吸引普通大众读者,汉英平行文本句法简明灵活,词汇多以普通词汇为主,将科学概念通俗化、趣味化,呈现口语化倾向,贴近生活,同时运用第一人称和第二人称拉近与读者的距离。

[**例3**] 中医强调:"邪之所凑,其气必虚,正气存内,邪不可干。"讲究养生,<u>正气强盛,即使流行病袭来,也可以减少发病;即使患病,病情也轻,康复也快</u>。

对比句: His doctor immediately admitted him to hospital where he was prescribed insulin, <u>an injectable treatment reserved for advanced cases</u>.

分析:汉语文本引用古文说明预防疾病的方法,并用现代文进行解释,以便于读者理解。同样,英语文本在提到"insulin"时,运用同位语结构"an injectable treatment reserved for advanced cases"对这一专业术语进行解释。

[**例4**] 我们每个家庭,都应开设<u>自己的健康银行</u>,舍得健康投资,这是最为划算的投资。

对比句 1: But for the glucose to get past the cells' membranes, it needs a "<u>key</u>" to get in. Insulin is that key.

对比句 2: A humane person loves people. This is an illustration to show that

Confucian humaneness may be equated to Christian godliness. Here humaneness means "love the people" while, for the equivalent Christian slogans, "God is love, and he who abides in love abides in God, and God abides in him."

分析：科普文章是内行写给外行看的，是科学和文学的结合，因此正式度要求不高。汉语例句和对比句 1 都运用比喻手法，使得抽象的理论和概念形象生动，使文章不再乏味枯燥，有助于科学知识的传播。对比句 2 把"儒家仁爱"和西方人熟悉的"基督教敬虔"联系起来，以最大限度地靠近目的语读者，使西方受众获得对异国文化的感性认识，增强对中医文化的认同。

二、篇章翻译的特点和策略

基于汉英科普读物在语篇结构和语言特点上的主要差异，我们对《治未病　大智慧》和《汪昂与〈汤头歌诀〉》进行翻译或翻译调整，以符合海外目标受众的阅读习惯和逻辑方式。

[例 5]　《治未病　大智慧》译文

Great Wisdom in Preventive Treatment

Dear Mr. Ren Zhiming,

① I've received your letter with great honor. You mentioned, in reading *Zhouyi* (*The Book of Changes*), you were enlightened by the sentence of "A man with vision can always foresee the potential misfortunes and take measures to prevent them from happening". I agree with you on this point. Measures should be employed in advance to avoid both social riots and human diseases.

②–⑤ Disease treatment should prioritize prevention. Treating a diseases from root means grasping the key of disease treatment. As early as 2000 years ago, our sages have warned people in *Huang Di Nei Jing* (*The Yellow Emperor's Internal Classic*) that "The sages usually pay less attention to the treatment of a disease, but more to its prevention. To resort to treatment when a disease has already occurred and resort to regulation when a disorder has already appeared is just like digging a well when one has been thirsty or casting weapons when a war has broken out. Wouldn't these actions be too late?" How wise are these words! Now you know that the best approach for disease treatment lies in prevention before it is developed. Similar idea has also been mentioned by Sun Simiao, China's King of Medicine in the Tang Dynasty (541–682), and Zhu Danxi, a renowned doctor in the Yuan Dynasty (1281 – 1358). Ancient sages even applied catchy rhymes to popularize the thoughts among general public. Just as an old disease-preventing rhyme vividly goes, "Overeating tasty food will lead to disease, and self-indulgence will result in misadventure. It would be better to strengthen prevention to nip the disease in the bud, rather than take drugs after it is fully developed." The modern folk proverb also says lively: "The dam should be built before a flood occurs, and a disease prevented before it occurs."

⑥⑦ The guiding philosophy of disease prevention advocated by the ancient sages is the most important concept for health maintenance. It is of great strategic significance to today's reality and mankind's future as well. In today's world, epidemics and infectious diseases such as influenza and viral hepatitis are posing a serious threat to our health, and dangerous killers such as stroke and myocardial infarction are claiming many lives. What should we do in the face of these two types of dangerous diseases? The fundamental solution is to mobilize the public to strengthen prevention at earliest time.

⑧-⑪ So how to prevent diseases? For one thing, we can strengthen prevention at mass level by hygiene strengthening, environment improvement and vaccine development. For another, we need to attach equal importance to practice health cultivation through preserving essence, qi and spirit, strengthening healthy qi, eliminating pathogenic qi to achieve individual prevention. Chinese medicine emphasizes that the accumulation of evils means the deficiency of qi; if there is sufficient healthy qi inside the body, evils cannot invade the body. To put it another way, if we practice health cultivation, we will strengthen our healthy qi and are less likely to catch epidemics, and even in case of getting diseases, we will exhibit slighter symptoms or recover faster. Chinese medicine also stresses that for those who can remain calm and avoid excessive desires and fantasies, their internal energies can circulate smoothly and freely, their mind can keep focused and concentrated, and thus they can avoid diseases. That is to say, health cultivation will help our body and mind in harmony, and thus decrease the occurrence of chronic diseases. Studies by WHO reveal that if we adopt a scientific, civilized and healthy lifestyle, and stick to the protocol of rational diet, appropriate amount of exercise, quitting smoking and limiting drinking, balanced mentality, we may cut the possibility of getting high blood pressure by 55%, stroke by

75%, diabetes by half, cancer by one third, and prolong our lives by 10 years.

⑫⑬ Today, the accessibility and affordability of health resources have become the public's focus of attention. It is true that this problem can be solved partly through medical reform and medical service, but they can only be uprooted through prioritizing disease prevention. While governments need to increase investment and emphasize disease prevention, individuals need to stick to health cultivation and disease prevention. Spending 10 yuan on disease prevention and health care may save 100 yuan of medical cost, and 1,000 or even 10,000 yuan of rescuing fee. Therefore, it is the most economical investment for each family to set up a health bank, just as indicated by the title of a report jointly issued by WHO and China's Ministry of Health in Beijing: *Preventing Chronic Diseases—A Vital Investment*. More importantly, we should take actions to prevent diseases before they occur based on adequate understanding of its importance. By following this way would individuals have less sufferings, families enjoy more happiness, and society become more harmonious. Here is "Ode to Preventative Treatment" to invite your pleasure:

Inaccessible health care and unaffordable medical costs

Make preventative treatment a wise choice

Stay away from disease to reduce medical expense

Without body and mind sufferings

Nor become families' encumbrance

Then society can become harmonious.

⑭ Mr. Ren, the profound idea of preventive treatment is a vivid manifestation of our predecessors' wisdom, and still serves as a guide for us to deal with diseases today through the millennia. At this point, I cannot help but exclaim: What an outstanding idea it is!

Best wishes for health and well-being!

Ma Youdu

分析：针对汉英科普读物语篇结构的不同特点，在翻译《治未病 大智慧》一文时，可对原文中较短但内容较为紧密的段落进行合并，并适当增添主题句，以更加符合西方读者的阅读习惯。此外,《治未病 大智慧》为增添文采,增强文章说服力,引经据典,大量引用中医药典籍文献和古代圣人先贤的语句,而这些内容有些是普通海外读者不需要了解的,或难以理解的,因此,译者需对该部分内容进行减译、改译或编译。

[**例6**] 《汪昂与〈汤头歌诀〉》翻译调整

Wang Ang and *Tang Tou Ge Jue (Versified Prescriptions)*

② In <u>Ming Dynasty (1368–1644)</u>, there appeared a famous physician named Wang Ang. ⑤ Since his childhood, Wang Ang loved poetry and literature. ⑥ After the fall of the Ming Dynasty, he started to learn medicine and read numerous medical books. ⑦ He found these medical books very boring, and decided to write his own books to attract more readers. ① He <u>also</u> found that with the development of prescription science, increasing number of medical formulas in specialized books brought great difficulties for beginners to comprehend and memorize. ③ <u>Therefore</u>, he compiled a book *Tang Tou Ge Jue (Versified Prescriptions)*, in which complex Chinese medicine prescriptions were adapted into rhymed songs suitable for recitation and memory.

④ For example, Wang Ang used six rhymed sentences to explain Si Jun Zi Tang (Four Gentlemen Decoction) <u>with its literal meaning as follows</u>: "There are four ingredients in this formula—Ren Shen (Radix et Rhizoma Ginseng), Bai Zhu (Rhizoma Atractylodis Macrocephalae), Fu Ling (Poria) and Gan Cao (Radix et Rhizoma Glycyrrhizae). This formula is called 'gentlemen' because of their equal dose and neutral property. If Ban Xia (Rhizoma Pinelliae) and Chen Pi (Pericarpium Citri Reticulatae) are added, this formula is called Liu Jun Zi Tang (Six Gentlemen Docoction), which acts to resolve phlegm, tonify qi and warm yang. If Ban Xia is removed, this formula is called Yi Gong San (Special Achievement Powder). In addition, when Mu Xiang (Radix Aucklandiae) and Sha Ren (Fructus Amomi) are added, this formula acts to circulate qi and warm the spleen and stomach."

⑧ The *Tang Tou Ge Jue* collected approximately 200 such versified formulas. The book was very popular after its publication, and it is still one of the necessary books for medical enlightenment. ⑨ Wang Ang has also been regarded as an important figure in promoting medical knowledge by later generations.

分析:改译按照"总—分—总"的篇章结构,将全文分为三段。第一段介绍汪昂学习中医药的背景和编写《汤头歌诀》的原因,第二段以"四君子汤"方歌为例,具体说明汪昂如何将复杂的中药药方编成押韵的歌诀以适合吟诵和记忆,第三段总结该书和汪昂对后世的影响。此外,改译在标题中添加"Tang Tou Ge Jue"的释译,正文中补充"Ming Dynasty"的起止时间,并在"四君子汤"方歌译文前添加"with its literal meaning as follows",说明下文是"四君子汤"方歌的字面翻译,而未体现原文押韵的特点,从而为海外读者提供必要的历史和文化背景。改译还增加了两个连接词"also"和"therefore",以加强行文连贯性,并将遗漏的第③、⑧和⑨全句或部分内容进行了补充,使得译文更加完整。

第三节　段落的翻译

译者在完成对语篇整体结构和内容的调整后,还须基于对段落命题之间逻辑关系的正确判断,根据海外读者的信息需求和阅读习惯,借鉴英语常规段落展开方式对段落进行调整,提升段落的连贯性和可读性。下文以《"生"的哲学》和其英译为例,讨论译文段落内部结构和内容调整。我们还将讨论汉语复合长句常见的逻辑关系和英译技巧。

一、段落翻译的特点和策略

[例1]　《"生"的哲学》与译文

分析:对照汉英文本发现,《"生"的哲学》的译文并没有和原文一一对应,而是在保留原文主要内容的前提下,对结构和内容进行了大幅度调整。原文通过引用孔子、孟子和其他儒家代表人物以及典籍的观点,阐述了"生"的哲学。第①~③句话引用孔子的话,提出"中国传统哲学是'生'的哲学";第④~⑥句阐述《易传》对孔子这一思想的发展,即"天地以'生'为道,以'生'为德";第⑦、⑧句进一步指出该思想的发展:"生"就是"仁","生"就是善;第⑨~⑫句引用儒家思想家的话对该观点进行说明;第⑬、⑭句进一步提出"儒家主张的'仁',不仅亲亲、爱人,而且从亲亲、爱人推广到爱天地万物";第⑮~㉑句中引用孟子和其他儒家代表人物的话对此加以阐述;最后第㉒句进行小结。

该段虽由浅入深分析了"生"的哲学,但在翻译过程中,如果不运用衔接手段,海外读者恐怕很难厘清句子之间繁杂的逻辑关系,加上众多儒家代表人物和名言,读者更难以抓住、理解主要内容。译文以海外读者信息需求和阅读习惯为出发点,对原文作了大量语序和内容调整。译文首先交代古代哲人对"生"思想的认识过程,在保留原文孔子和《易传》引言的基础上,考虑到孟子的影响以及海外读者对孟子的熟悉度,将孟子的例子提前,并增译孟子的背景知识。第⑦句起到承上启下的作用,概述后代的儒家思想家都继承孔子和《易传》的思想,强调人的仁心、善心。第⑦句后一句是增译,概括说明宋朝许多知名儒家学者对该观点的传承,并用"for example"显化句间的逻辑关系。列举宋代知名学者的观点时进行了删减,只保留原文中代表性较强的人物和引言,即第⑨、⑪、⑰句。第⑬句增译"We can see from their thoughts that"总结全文,并改用第一人称以拉近和读者的距离,增强译文的亲切感。可见,调整过的译文充分考虑了海外读者的知识背景和阅读习惯,逻辑清楚,连贯性强,具有很强的可读性。

二、句子翻译的特点和策略

从翻译角度来看,汉语复合长句的逻辑关系分为总分、因果、并列、铺垫—主旨及主旨—补充关系等等。在翻译过程中,译者须准确分析原文句间逻辑关系,再运用适当语言策略译出。

1. 因果关系

[例2] ① 相传西汉文帝时,湖南郴州有一位名医叫苏耽,② 他医术精湛,好助人为乐,人称"苏仙翁"。①

译文:① During the reign of Emperor Wen of Han, there was a well-known physician named Su Dan in Chenzhou, Hunan Province. ② He was called "Su Xian Weng (immortal Su)" because of his medical skills and readiness to help others.

分析:汉语的因果关系多隐含在语境中,英语的因果关系既有隐形性表达,又有显性表达。在英译过程中,须将汉语隐含的因果关系显性化。例句第②句的"医术精湛,好助人为乐"和"人称'苏仙翁'"是因果关系,但是为隐形表达,英译时需用"because of"显化这种关系。

2. 铺垫—主旨关系和主旨—补充关系

[例3] ① 益以夏陈名六君,② 祛痰补气阳虚饵。②

---

① 选自:"画说中医药文化"丛书编委会. 中医史画[M]. 北京:中国轻工业出版社,2018: 62 - 63.

② 选自:"画说中医药文化"丛书编委会. 中医史画[M]. 北京:中国轻工业出版社,2018: 124 - 125.

译文：① By adding Ban Xia (Rhizoma Pinelliae) and Chen Pi (Pericarpium Citri Reticulatae)， this formula is called Liu Jun Zi Tang (Six Gentlemen Docoction)， ② which acts to resolve phlegm, tonify qi and warm yang.

分析：铺垫—主旨关系包括递进、转折、假设、背景—主题、条件—结论、虚写—实写等关系,它们都遵循"次要—主要"的逻辑关系,对于铺垫部分的次要信息,可以用定语从句、同位语、前置独立结构、插入语、标点符号等。相反,体现主旨—补充关系的句子在翻译时,补充成分可以用独立结构、非限制性定语从句或其他结构翻译。本例的主要信息是"名六君","益以夏陈"说明"六君"的构成,"祛痰补气阳虚饵"说明"六君"的功效,译文通过介词短语和定语从句,清楚地表达出句子中的"次要—主要—次要"关系。

3. 连动关系

[例4]　① 他把羊肉、辣椒和祛寒药材放在锅里熬煮,② 然后将羊肉、药物捞出切碎,③ 用面皮包成耳朵样的"娇耳",④ 煮熟后分给求药的人每人两只"娇耳"、一大碗肉汤。①

原译：① He put and decocted mutton, pepper and other cold-dispelling medicines in the pot, ② then took the meat and medicines out and got them chopped, ③ and made ear-shaped food with pastry wrapper. ④ Each one who sought for treatment would get two Jiao Er and a bowl of meat soup.

改译：① He began the process by putting mutton, pepper and other cold-dispelling medicines in a pot and decocted them together. ②③ After taking mutton and medicine out and chopping them, he wrapped the filling into flour crust to make ear-shaped Jiao'er. ④ Each one who sought for treatment would get two boiled Jiao'ers and a bowl of meat soup.

分析：连动关系是一个施事主语带三个以上的谓语动词。翻译时可以在几个动词之间或最后加上"and""then"等衔接词;也可以在几个连动动词中选取一个或几个作为补充、背景,用现在分词表示,其他的数个或一个作为突出、前景,用基本时态表示;还可以用"where""before""when"等连词引导的从句表示后续动作。该句描述了"放""熬煮""捞出""切碎""包"等做"娇耳"的一系列动作,原译第①、②、③句用

---

①　选自："画说中医药文化"丛书编委会. 药膳趣画[M]. 北京：中国轻工业出版社,2018：106 – 107.

"then""and"等词语表达出动作过程,但语言略显单调,句间关系也不够紧密。改译后第①句增加了"began the process by"统领下面动作,将第②、③句浓缩为一句,用"after""to"两个介词清晰地表示出动作的连贯性,并将"用面皮包成耳朵样的'娇耳'"改译为"wrapped the filling into flour crust to make ear-shaped Jiao'er",交代"娇耳"这一中国特色食品的由来。

4. 并列关系

[例5] ① 中医四大经典在这一时期集中涌现:②《黄帝内经》和《难经》为中医理论之源,③《神农本草经》为本草学之祖,④ 张仲景的《伤寒杂病论》则开启了临床辨证施治之端。①

译文:① This period witnessed the emergence of four major classics in traditional Chinese medicine—*Huang Di Nei Jing, Nan Jing, Shen Nong Ben Cao Jing* and *Shang Han Za Bing Lun*. ② The first two has been treated as the fundamental doctrinal source for Chinese medicine. ③ *Shen Nong Ben Cao Jing* has been regarded as the first book on Chinese herbs. ④ *Shang Han Za Bing Lun* by Zhang Zhongjing initiated the treatment protocols according to syndrome differentiation.

分析:译者先在第①句补充中医四大经典名称,然后分别在第②、③、④句列出每部经典的卓越之处。我们也可以用分号或"and"将原②、③、④句合为一句,加强并列关系。

第四节 词语的翻译

中医药科普读物会经常出现中医药术语和有关中国历史文化的特色词汇,本节讨论如何灵活运用直译、意译、释译、省译、增译等翻译技巧,用通俗易懂的语言传播中医药知识和文化。

一、中医药术语翻译

中医药术语翻译既要科学性强,又要具有可读性,经常采用的翻译技巧包括直

---

① 选自:"画说中医药文化"丛书编委会. 中医史画[M]. 北京:中国轻工业出版社,2018:34-35.

译、音译加注释、意译、释译等。

[**例1**] 如"四君子汤":"四君子汤中和义,参术茯苓甘草比……"。①

原译: Take Si Jun Zi Tang（Four Gentlemen Decoction）for example . . . This formula is called "gentlemen" because of their equal dose and neutral property.

改译1: Take Si Jun Zi Tang（Four Gentlemen Decoction）for example . . . This formula is called "four gentlemen" of herbal medicine because the four herbs in this formula are mild in nature and blend well together in tonifying the qi.

改译2: Take Decoction of Four Mild Drugs for example . . .

分析: 原译采用拼音加直译的译法,并增加释译"This formula is called 'gentlemen' because of their equal dose and neutral property",使译文与原文基本取得内容与形式的统一,但对"四君子汤"内涵的解释可以更加深入。"四君子汤"完整释译为:

In traditional Chinese culture it was common to refer to four important things that were harmonious as a group and not given to extremes as the "four gentlemen" or the "four noblemen" after the Confucian term for a person who exhibits ideal behavior. The four herbs in this formula are mild in nature and blend well together in tonifying the qi. They are therefore called the "four gentlemen" of herbal medicine.②

该释译虽达意,但直接放在译文中显得冗长,我们可将释译拆开,巧妙地插入译文中,如改译1所示。但是,添加释译难免影响语篇的连贯性,在这种情况下,我们可意译,如改译2所示。比喻是中医词语修辞的一大特色,"四君子汤"就是比喻描写,读起来带有浓厚的文学色彩。但科普读物属于科技文体,这种文体旨在阐述理论、思想和成果,在表达上要求语言简洁、逻辑清晰,一般不用带有感情色彩的词汇。因此遇到这种词汇,意译也是一种不错的选择。

[**例2**] 得道成仙本属虚幻,但这一传说却反映了人们对祛病保健的美好愿望和良医大家的仰慕之情。自此,中医药史上就有了"橘井泉香"的佳话,后人也用其形容医术高超、治病救人的中医。③

原译: This mythical story indicated the people's wishes to ward off diseases and

---

① 选自:"画说中医药文化"丛书编委会. 中医史画[M]. 北京:中国轻工业出版社,2018:124-125.

② 选自:郑玲. 中医英语译写教程[M] 北京:中国古籍出版社,2013:30.

③ 选自:"画说中医药文化"丛书编委会. 中医史画[M]. 北京:中国轻工业出版社,2018:62-63.

admiration for doctors. The story of <u>Ju Jing Quan Xiang (tangerine leaves and well water)</u> has become a well-told tale in the history of traditional Chinese medicine.

改译：This mythical story reflects people's wishes to ward off diseases and admiration for doctors, and therefore become a well-told tale in the history of traditional Chinese medicine. <u>Ju Jing Quan Xiang (tangerine leaves and well water)</u> is used <u>to refer to the highly skilled doctors who are capable of treating and saving patients with Chinese medicine.</u>

分析："橘井泉香"采用的也是比喻描写,原译运用了音译和直译策略,改译通过补译原文中最后一句"后人也用其形容医术高超、治病救人的中医"进行必要释译,帮助海外读者更好地理解其中医文化内涵。

二、文化负载词翻译

在翻译文化负载词时,译者需要具有强烈的受众意识,根据受众内外有别的原则,采取深化或浅化的翻译策略,对于海外读者不感兴趣的内容,或有损于国家形象的内容要果断删去。反之,如果特色词汇体现中医药传统文化的核心概念,或对译文的连贯性至关重要,则需进行必要的注解和解释,以加强读者的理解,促进中医药文化的对外传播。

[例3] <u>孟子说:"亲亲而仁民,仁民而爱物。"</u>①

译文：Mencius (<u>c. 372 - 289 BC</u>), <u>a great Confucian scholar who lived just over 100 years after Confucius,</u> said, " (One should) love one's family, love the people, and love all living things in the world. "②

分析：译文运用增译法,补充孟子的生辰,并说明孟子是继孔子之后一位伟大的儒家学者,从而增强孟子引言的权威性。海外读者对这些中国读者耳熟能详的人物可能比较陌生,如不加以注解,读者可能难以领会引言的重要性,也会影响语篇的连贯性,因此很有必要进行深化翻译。

[例4] 汪昂出生在明朝末年,早年爱好诗文,<u>明朝灭亡后不愿为清廷效忠</u>,才弃儒学医。③

---

① 选自: 叶朗,朱良志. 中国文化读本[M]. 北京: 外语教学与研究出版社,2016: 60 - 61.

② 选自: Ye L, Zhu L Z. *Insights into Chinese Culture*[M]. Beijing: Foreign Language Teaching and Research Press, 2008: 34 - 35.

③ 选自:"画说中医药文化"丛书编委会. 中医史画[M]. 北京: 中国轻工业出版社,2018: 124 - 125.

译文：Born in the later years of Ming Dynasty, Wang Ang loved poetry and literature. After the fall of the Ming Dynasty, he started to learn medicine and read numerous medical books.

分析：译者省译了"明朝灭亡后不愿为清廷效忠"一句。如翻译此句，海外读者很难理解汪昂在明朝灭亡后不愿为清廷效忠的原因，加注解会影响语篇的连贯性，并可能会导致读者的误解。因此，在不影响全篇主题的前提下，略去此句是非常合适的选择。

第五节　翻译练习与任务

一、翻译练习

1. 以下两段分别选自 *Contemporary Introduction to Chinese Medicine—In Comparison with Western Medicine*（《打开中医之门：针对西方读者的中医导论》）和 *The Web That Has No Weaver—Understanding Chinese Medicine*（《无人编织的网：理解中医》），对比分析术语翻译方法和策略上的差异，并分析原因。

（1）The spleen (-zang) and the stomach coordinate in digestion and assimilation. Both organs are regarded as the "source of regenerating qi and blood" and the "root of acquired constitution." Their functions are often opposite in direction: ... The two organs also have other opposite functional properties, e. g. , the intolerance of dryness by the stomach vs intolerance of dampness by the spleen (-zang), the innermost location of the spleen (-zang) (the extreme yin of yin organs with no passage to the outside) vs. the outermost location of the stomach (the organ that receives food and drink through the mouth from outside). It is those opposite functional properties that make the stomach and spleen (-zang) complement and restrain each other, so that a harmonious coordination can be maintained. Pathologically, the stomach and the spleen (-zang) are often involved simultaneously.

（2）The Stomach like Dampness and is sensitive to Dryness, while the opposite is true of the Spleen. Thus, Deficient Yin of the Stomach is a common pattern, while Dampness disharmony is typical of the Spleen.

2. 将下面选自《中国日报》的介绍德国医史学家文树德教授(Prof. Paul U. Unschuld)的短文译为英文。

5 月 26 日，是《本草纲目》入选 UNESCO 世界记忆名录 10 周年。这背后有一位德国人默默做了大量工作，而且近 20 年来，他一直在努力做一件事——把《本草纲目》翻译成英文。他就是文树德先生。

文树德先生 1943 年生，医史学家。专攻中、欧医学及生命科学比较史，尤擅长医学思想史、伦理史研究，1969 年开始研习中医药学，1986 年任慕尼黑大学医史研究所所长。他是首位采用严格的文献学和史学方法，将中国古代医学经典著作翻译成英语的西方人。

"我每天八个小时坐在这里翻译《本草纲目》的内容。现在快 78 岁了，我希望 80 岁以前可以完成《本草纲目》的翻译。"文先生说。

"从实用性角度来看，《本草纲目》既让各国读者知道中国传统的药物知识是多么广泛，也能促使读者了解古代植物知识，还能发展现代新型药物，这是很重要的。"

"我为什么尊敬李时珍？第一，他的知识来源广泛，从贩夫走卒到儒释道，包罗万象。他怎么可以有这样一个 open mind（开放心态）！"文树德先生说。

"第二个是他的 flexibility（灵活性）。他不仅提自己的医案，而且有很多别人的有效的、成功的医案。"

"现在西医的药物，70% 有植物的基础，70% 现在最常用的药物有流传下来的植物的基础。温故知新，把中医中药与西医西药和现代科学结合在一起，可以发展现代医学，造福全人类。"

二、翻译任务

1. 以下这封信选自《奇妙中医药：家庭保健顾问》一书。以小组的形式将此封信译为英文，讨论翻译过程中在语篇、段落和词语层面做的翻译调整及原因，以及采取的翻译策略。

健康·长寿·快乐

任智明先生：

捧读来信，特别高兴。酒逢知己千杯少，说话投机自然多。面对你的来信，遥望窗外的星空，不禁浮想联翩，许多话都想对你诉说。梳理一下思路，最想说的还是咱们的中华养生文化。

中医药养生，既讲医理，又富哲理，而且文采飞扬。你看看《证治百问》的这段话：

"人之性情最喜畅快,形神最宜焕发,如此刻刻有长春之性,时时有长生之情,不惟却病,可以永年。"说得多么好啊! 仅仅 38 个字,就把健康、长寿、快乐刻画得活灵活现,医理之中寓哲理,细细品味,妙趣深深。人要健康,全靠身心和谐,形神焕发,特别要做到性情畅快,这就是永葆青春的妙诀,既可健康不病,又可延年益寿,还能天天快乐。要想延年益寿,离不开健康,要想天天快乐,更是离不开健康。我还想特别强调:"大千世界,以人为本,人生幸福,健康为本。"拥有健康,才能创造幸福,也只有拥有健康,才能享受幸福。印度《五卷书》说得好:"在地球上没有什么收获比得上健康。"阿拉伯谚语也强调指出:"有健康的人,便有希望。有希望的人,便有一切。"

健康是事业的本钱,拥有健康,才能助你建功立业、发家致富、成名成家。如果丧失健康,即使一时成功,最后还是以失败告终。世界卫生组织总干事马勒博士说得明白:"健康不是一切,但失去健康便失去一切。"古希腊著名哲学家赫拉克列特说得最为深刻:"如果没有健康,智慧不能发挥,文化无法施展,知识无法利用,就没有力量去战斗和创造财富。"

古今中外的这些格言警语,何等精彩,是生存智慧的结晶,是极为珍贵的精神财富,给我们启迪,让我们深思。

健康这么重要,那么怎样才算健康呢?

有人说,没有病就叫健康,这种看法不全面。有人说,身体好就叫健康,这种看法也不全面。

真正的健康,至少要符合三条标准。世界卫生组织(WHO)将健康概括为这样一句话:"健康就是身体上、心理上和社会适应上的完美状态。"后来,进一步的研究表明,只符合以上三条标准,并不完美,还必须再加上一条重要的标准——道德健康。

我的看法是,真正完美的健康,应当包括五条标准:① 身体健康;② 心理健康;③ 道德健康;④ 人与大自然适应;⑤ 人与社会适应。应当做到三个和谐:① 身心和谐;② 人天和谐;③ 人际和谐。用一句话来概括:"健康就是身体健康、心理健康、道德健康、人天适应、人际和谐的完美状态。"

要想延年益寿,离不开健康;要想天天快乐,更是离不开健康。如果只是寿命活得长,身体不健康,病痛缠身,也就没有多少乐趣可言。苏联哈列斯基说得好:"如果一个人只忙着同疾病作斗争,那长寿的乐趣也就不大了!"现实中的例子,确实是这样。有的人年过八旬,有的人活到九十高龄,但却没有健康,长期卧床,生活不能自理,吃喝拉撒全靠别人照料,一年四季病痛不断,甚至重病缠身,度日如年。这样的长寿,究竟有多少乐趣可言呢? 所以,我们要争取的是健康的长寿,既不增加家庭的拖累,也不成为社会的负担,而且可以充分发挥自己的余热,贡献于家庭,服务于社会,并从中享受老有所为的快乐。

人生的幸福,不仅寓于寿而康,而且在于乐而康,只有这样,我们才能真正做到"多活些年,多做些事,多享些福"。

智明先生,我们崇尚健康,我们追求长寿,我们更要品味快乐。人生一世,从小到老为的就是快乐,为大众创造快乐,自己也从中不断地品味快乐,这才是延年益寿永葆青春的真谛。还是前贤说得好:"人之性情最喜畅快,形神最宜焕发,如此刻刻有长春之性,时时有长生之情。"妙哉斯言!

祝健康　长寿　快乐

马有度

2. 选择一篇古往今来中医大师或海内外中医著名翻译家的故事并译为英文,思考他们所体现的医者仁心、大医精诚的精神,孜孜不倦、精益求精的科研精神,或深厚的家园情怀和爱国主义精神。

三、扩展阅读

［1］Xie Z F, Xie F. *Contemporary Introduction to Chinese Medicine—In Comparison with Western Medicine*［M］. Beijing: Foreign Language Press, 2010.

［2］Kaptchuk T J. *The Web That Has No Weaver—Understanding Chinese Medicine*［M］. New York: McGraw-Hill, 2000.

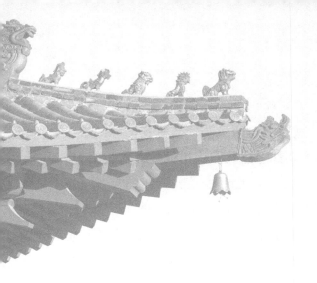

第六章
中成药说明书英译

中成药说明书是载明中成药药品重要信息的法定文件,是医护人员和患者了解药品的重要途径。高质量的英译版中成药说明书是中药走向世界的敲门砖,在中药的推广过程中占据着重要的地位。中成药说明书英译不仅要传达医学信息,让海外消费者了解和熟悉药品的药理作用、用法、用量、适应证、禁忌等,而且要能激发海外消费者的购买欲,使其最终采取购买该药品的行动,以此促进产品在海外的销售以及中医药文化的对外传播。刘明等(2016:118-119)对2002—2016年间发表的57篇有关中药说明书翻译的论文进行了分类统计,结果显示,说明书英译主要问题是药品名称翻译混乱、功效语语句欠妥、英译标准不统一、结构内容缺失、可读性差等,其他问题还有望文生义、错译漏译、语法错误、翻译死板、中式思维严重等。本章聚焦说明书语篇、功效语以及药名和其他术语的英译,基于平行文本对比分析,提取和归纳翻译策略,促进实现译文的预期交际目的,提升译文的质量和传播力。

第一节 语料导入

我国的中成药市场产品中,用于出口的主要是抗感冒类、抗病毒类以及清热解毒类的药品,因此本章选取治疗呼吸类疾病的中成药中英文说明书作为分析语料。语料分为两组,一组是10份内地中成药产品的中文说明书(以下简称"内地说明书")和原译,主要选自涂雯(2018:25)建立的中成药中英文说明书语料库,包括《健民咽喉片说明书》《急支糖浆说明书》《咳喘丸说明书》《藿香正气胶囊说明书》等。第二组是10份香港中成药产品的中英文说明书(以下简称"香港说明书"),选自香港京都念慈菴、位元堂、余仁生等中药公司的网站。这些公司的中药产品得到国际权威认证,英文说明书比较适合作为参考语料,包括《京都念慈菴蜜炼川贝枇杷膏说明书》《清嗓饮说明书》《小柴胡汤说明书》《藿香正气散颗粒说明书》《养阴丸说明书》《银翘散颗粒说明书》等等。此外,选取1篇西药说明书"NASAL DECONGESTANT"(《鼻腔减充血片说明书》)作为语篇层面分析语料。本节仅列出用于语篇分析的语料,段落和词语分析语料在第三节、第四节分别呈现,本节不再列出。

一、中文语料(包括原译)

1.《健民咽喉片说明书》

健民®咽喉片

鄂卫准字(90)1325号

本品根据中医验方"玄麦甘桔汤"等方剂综合研制,用于急慢性咽喉炎及发音器官的保健。经316例临床验证,治疗急慢性咽喉炎总有效率为95.9%,经武汉卫生部门鉴定,批准生产。

本品为纯中药制剂,其配方含:玄参、生地、麦冬、桔梗、胖大海、板蓝根、藏青果等十三种中药。经药理研究实验证明:本品能扩张微血管、改善微循环,增加唾液及唾液蛋白分泌,减轻炎性组织所致的疼痛,对急性炎症的渗出和水肿有明显的抑制作用。本品对甲型链球菌、乙型溶血性链球菌、金黄色葡萄球菌及肺炎双球菌、脑膜炎双球菌、大肠杆菌等有抑制作用。

本品在含化过程中,药物缓慢释放,通过咽喉黏膜溶解吸收,对整个机体有清热泻火之功效。其疗效优于其他含片,且无毒副作用。

中国武汉健民药业(集团)股份有限公司

武汉市健民制药厂

地址:武汉市汉阳市鹦鹉大道384号

JIAN MIN YAN HOU PIAN

(Tablet in Mouth)

Authorized Registration No. HBMP (90) 1325

JIAN MIN YAN HOU PIAN is based on "xuan mai gan jie decoction," proved recipe from traditional Chinese medicine, is indicated for the acute and chronic pharyngitis and benefits the voice organs. The effective rate is as high as 95.9% proved by the clinical study in 316 cases. It has been approved by Wuhan Hygienic Bureau for the production.

This drug is a pure Chinese herbal preparation. It contains Radix Scrophulariae, Radix rehmanniae, Radix Isatidis, etc., thirteen kinds of drugs. It is proved by pharmacologic test that it can dilate capillary, improve microcirculation, increase saliva and saliva protein, alleviate patients' pain caused by inflammatory tissue, and suppress seepage and edema caused by acute inflammation. It is proved by bacteriostatic test that it can suppress the growth of B-hemolytic streptococcus, staphylococcus aurous, diplococcus pneumonlae, meningococcus and colibacillus.

This drug can clear pharynx, moisten throat to promote the production of body fluid, detoxify and purge the fire. Its action is better than other tablets in mouth, no any side and toxic effect.

China Wuhan Jianmin Pharmaceutical (Groups) Co. Ltd.

Wuhan Jianmin Pharmaceutical Factory

Add: No. 384 Ying Wu Ave.

Hanyang, Wuhan, China

2.《急支糖浆说明书》

急支糖浆说明书

请仔细阅读说明书并按照使用或在药师指导下购买和使用。

[**药品名称**]

通用名称：急支糖浆

汉语拼音：Jizhi Tangjiang

[**成　　份**]鱼腥草、金荞麦、四季青、麻黄、紫菀、前胡、枳壳、甘草。辅料为蔗糖、苯甲酸、山梨酸钾。

[**性　　状**]本品为棕褐色的黏稠液体;味甜、微苦。

[**功能主治**]清热化痰,宣肺止咳。用于外感风热所致的咳嗽,症见发热、恶寒、胸膈满闷、咳嗽咽痛;急性支气管炎、慢性支气管炎急性发作见上述证候者。

[**用法用量**]口服,一次20~30毫升,一日3~4次;儿童一岁以内一次5毫升,一岁至三岁一次7毫升,三岁至七岁一次10毫升,七岁以上一次15毫升,一日3~4次。

[**不良反应**]尚不明确。

[**禁　　忌**]尚不明确。

[**注意事项**]1. 忌烟、酒及辛辣、生冷、油腻食物。2. 不宜在服药期间同时服用滋补性中药。3. 支气管扩张、肺脓疡、肺心病、肺结核患者出现咳嗽时应去医院就诊。4. 高血压、心脏病患者慎用。糖尿病患者及有肝病、肾病等慢性病严重患者应在医师指导下服用。5. 儿童、孕妇、哺乳期妇女、年老体弱者应在医师指导下服用。6. 服药期间,若患者发热体温超过38.5℃,或出现喘促气急者,或咳嗽加重、痰量明显增多者应去医院就诊。7. 服药3天症状无缓解,应去医院就诊。8. 对本品过敏者禁用,过敏体质者慎用。9. 本品性状发生改变时禁止使用。10. 儿童必须在成人监护下使用。11. 请将本品放在儿童不能接触的地方。12. 如正在使用其他药品,使用本品前请咨询医师或药师。13. 运动员慎用。

[**药物相互作用**]如与其他药物同时使用可能会发生药物相互作用,详情咨询医师或药师。

[**贮　　藏**]密封。

[**包　　装**]聚酯塑料瓶包装,每瓶装300毫升。

[**有 效 期**]36个月

[**执行标准**]《中国药典》2015年版一部

[**批准文号**]国药准字Z33020852

[**说明书修订日期**]2016年04月25日

[**生产企业**]企业名称：太极集团浙江东方制药有限公司

ACUTE BRONCHITIS SYRUP

Composition:

Herba Houttuyniae cordata Thumb, Fagopyrum cymosum, Ilicis purpureae Hassk, Herba Ephedrae, Radix Asteris, Radix Peucedami, Fructus auranti, Radix Glycyrrhizae and adjuvants: Sucrose, Benzoic acid, Potassium sorbate.

Actions and Indications:

Clearing heat and transform phlegm: diffuse the lung and suppress cough. Use for the treatment due to the external contraction of wind and fever with symptoms of an aversion to cold with fever, fullness and oppression in the chest and diaphragm, cough and sore pharynx, acute bronchitis, and acute attack of chronic bronchitis with the above mentioned symptoms.

Dosage and Administration:

Orally, 20 – 30 mL at a time, 3 or 4 times a day; for children under one year, 5 mL each time; 1 to 3 years, 7 mL each time; 3 to 7 years, 10 mL each time and above 7 years, 15 mL at a time, 3 or 4 times a day.

Adverse drug reaction:

No any study report available.

Contraindication:

No any study report available.

Caution:

Carefully read the Directions of Use.

Storage:

Keep tightly close.

Package: Packaged in plastic bottle, 300 mL/bottle/box.

3.《京都念慈菴蜜炼川贝枇杷膏说明书》

京都念慈菴蜜炼川贝枇杷膏说明书

请仔细阅读说明书并按照使用或在药师指导下购买和使用

［**药品名称**］

通用名称：京都念慈菴蜜炼川贝枇杷膏

汉语拼音：Jingdu Niancian Milian Chuanbei Pipa Gao

［**成　　份**］川贝母、枇杷叶、南沙参、茯苓、化橘红、桔梗、法半夏、五味子、款冬花、远志、苦杏仁、生姜、甘草、杏仁水、薄荷脑,辅料为蜂蜜、麦芽糖、糖浆。

［**性　　状**］本品为棕褐色黏稠的半流体;具杏仁香气,味甜,辛凉。

［**功能主治**］润肺化痰、止咳平喘、护喉利咽、生津补气、调心降火。本品适用于伤风咳嗽、痰稠、痰多气喘、咽喉干痒及声音嘶哑。

［**用法用量**］口服,成人每日3次,每次一汤勺,儿童酌减。

［**不良反应**］本品可能引起皮疹、瘙痒、腹泻、腹痛、恶心等。

［**禁　　忌**］糖尿病患者忌用。

［**注意事项**］

1. 忌烟、酒及辛辣、生冷、油腻食物。

2. 患有肝病、肾病等慢性疾病严重者应在医生指导下服用。

3. 服药一周病情无改善,或服药期间症状加重者,应停止服用,去医院就诊。

4. 本品性状发生改变时禁止使用。

5. 儿童必须在成人监护下使用。

6. 请将本品放在儿童不能接触的地方。

7. 如正在使用其他药品,使用本品前请咨询医师或药师。

8. 孕妇、哺乳期妇女、儿童、老人等应在医师指导下使用。

[**药物相互作用**]如与其他药物同时使用可能会发生药物相互作用,详情咨询医师或药师。

[**贮　藏**]密封,置阴凉处。(不超过20℃)

[**包　装**]玻璃瓶装,每瓶装300毫升。

[**有 效 期**]36个月。

[**执行标准**]进口药品注册标准JZ20160002

[**批准文号**]医药产品注册证号ZC20160006

[**说明书修订日期**]2016年4月13日

[**生产公司**]

公司名称:京都念慈菴总厂有限公司

生产地址:香港新界元朗元朗工业邨宏利街50号京都念慈菴中心

电话号码:(00852)2438-9988

传真号码:(00852)2407-6269

网址:www. ninjiom. com

[**中国大陆联络处**]广东伟沂贸易有限公司

NIN JIOM PEI PA KOA

(Traditional Chinese Herbal Coughs Syrup)

Indications

Nin Jiom Pei Pa Koa is formulated from Chinese herbal ingredients and plant extracts together with honey and sugar syrups and has a pleasant taste. It provides temporary relief of coughs and sore throat associated with common cold, influenza or similar ailments. Nin Jiom Pei Pa Koa is effective for the temporary relief of the symptoms of bronchial cough and loss of voice.

Dosage

Adults:　　3 times a day.

　　　　　One tablespoon a time.

Children:　3 times a day.

　　　　　Dosage to be reduced according to age.

Ingredients

Tendrilleaf Fritillary Bulb	Common Coltsfoot Flower
Loquat Leaf	Thinleaf Milkwort Root
Fourleaf ladybell Root	Bitter Apricot Seed
Indian Bread	Fresh Ginger
Pummelo Peel	Liquorice Root
Platycodon Root	Menthol
Prepared Pinellia Tuber	Honey
Chinese Magnoliavine Fruit	Maltose
Snakeground Seed	Syrup

二、英文语料

NASAL DECONGESTANT(《鼻腔减充血片说明书》)

NASAL DECONGESTANT—pseudoephedrine HCl tablet, film coated

L. N. K. International, Inc.

Disclaimer: Most OTC drugs are not reviewed and approved by FDA, however, they may be marketed if they comply with applicable regulations and policies. FDA has not evaluated whether this product complies.

Quality Plus 44 - 112

Active ingredient (in each tablet)

Pseudoephedrine HCl 30 mg

Purpose

Nasal decongestant

Uses

—temporarily relieves nasal congestion due to the common cold, fever or other upper respiratory allergies

—temporarily relieves sinus congestion and pressure

Warnings

Do not use

if you are now taking a prescription monoamine oxidase inhibitor (MAOI) (certain drugs for depression, psychiatric or emotional conditions, or Parkinson's disease), or for

2 weeks after stopping the MAOI drug. If you do not know if your prescription drug contains MAOI, ask a doctor or pharmacist before taking this product.

Ask a doctor before use if you have

—diabetes

—heart disease

—high blood pressure

—thyroid disease

—difficulty in urination due to enlargement of the prostate gland

When using this product

Do not exceed recommended dosage.

Stop use and ask a doctor if

—nervousness, dizziness, or sleeplessness occur

—symptoms do not improve within 7 days or occur with fever

If pregnant or breast-feeding,

Ask a health professional before use.

Keep out of reach of children.

In case of overdose, get medical help or contact a Poison Control Center (1 - 800 - 222 - 1222) right away.

Directions

Adults and children 12 and older	Take 2 tablets every 4 – 6 hours; do not take more than 8 tablets within 24 hours.
Children aged 6 to 11 years	Take 1 tablet every 4 – 6 hours; do not take more than 4 tablets within 24 hours.
Children under 6 years	Do not use.

Other information

—**each tablet contains:** calcium 15 mg

—**TAMPER EVIDENT: DO NOT USE IF OUTER PACKAGE IS OPENED OR BLISTER IS TORN OR BROKEN**

—store at 25℃ (77℉); excursions permitted between 15℃-30℃ (59℉-86℉)

—see end flap for expiration date and lot number

Inactive ingredients

croscarmellose sodium, dibasic calcium phosphate dihydrate, FD&C red #40 aluminum lake, FD&C yellow #6 aluminum lake, hypromellose, magnesium stearate, microcrystalline cellulose, polydextrose, polyethylene glycol, silicon dioxide, titanium dioxide, triacetin

Questions or comments?

1 – 800 – 426 – 9391

TAMPER EVIDENT: DO NOT USE IF PACKAGE IS OPENED OR IF BLISTER UNIT IS TORN, BROKEN OR SHOWS ANY SIGNS OF TAMPERING

Distributed by **LNK INTERNATIONAL, INC.**

60 Arkay Drive,

Hauppauge, NY 11788

第二节　篇章的翻译

一、篇章对比分析

1. 纲要式结构

药品说明书的结构比较固定,结构语一般包括药品名称(Drug)、主要成分(Composition)、性状(Description)、功能主治/适用症(Indications)/作用与用途(Actions and Uses)、用法用量(Administration and Dosage)、不良反应(Adverse Reactions)/副作用(Side Effects;Side-effects)、禁忌(Contraindications)、注意事项(Precautions)、药物相互作用(Pharmacological Actions)/临床药理(Clinical Pharmacology)/毒理学(Toxicology)、贮藏(Storage)、包装(Package)、有效期/失效期(Expiry Date)、批准文号和生产公司(Manufacturer)。

对比分析发现,《急支糖浆说明书》《京都念慈菴蜜炼川贝枇杷膏说明书》和"NASAL DECONGESTANT"的结构语都比较完整,而《健民咽喉片说明书》采取分段表述的形式,由于每段内容包含一个或多个主题,也没有结构语,语篇结构显得不清晰,主要信息不突出,有必要进行改译。

2. 体现样式

在语言表达上,药品说明书一般运用正式用语、专业术语和第三人称以保证内容客观、科学、准确,该特点在汉英平行文本中都得到了体现。值得注意的是,《京都念慈菴蜜炼川贝枇杷膏说明书》出现了"pleasant"等表明个人态度和情感的评价语,以达到拉近与读者的距离、增强译文的感染性的目的。

外观设计也是说明书体现样式不可忽略的重要组成部分,一份外观醒目、排版悦目的说明书能使读者快速找到所需信息,提升读者的阅读感受。《急支糖浆说明书》原译中"性状""注意事项"等重要内容没有译出,过度简化。在排版上,由于缺乏对海外受众阅读感受的充分考虑,每部分内容只采用了单一的文字形式,不免会加重读者的阅读负担。平行文本"NASAL DECONGESTANT"以加粗加黑、变化字体、分行单列、图表等多种形式突出显示说明书的重要信息。

二、篇章翻译的特点和策略

[例1] 《健民咽喉片说明书》英译纲要式结构调整

JIAN MIN YAN HOU PIAN

(Throat Tablets)

Authorized Registration No. HBMP (90) 1325

Composition

Thirteen kinds of drugs including Radix Scrophulariae, Radix Rehmanniae, Radix Isatidis, etc.

Actions & Indications

JIAN MIN YAN HOU PIAN is based on Xuan Mai Gan Jie Decoction, a proved formula of traditional Chinese medicine. It can clear pharynx, moisten throat to promote the production of body fluid, detoxify and purge the fire, and is effective for the temporary relief of acute and chronic pharyngitis symptoms.

Adverse Reactions

No side and toxic effects.

Clinical Pharmacology

Approved by Wuhan Hygienic Bureau for the production, this drug has the effective rate as high as 95.9% as proved by the clinical study in 316 cases. Pharmacologic test proves that it can dilate capillary, improve microcirculation, increase saliva and saliva protein, alleviate patients' pain caused by inflammatory tissue, and suppress seepage and edema caused by acute inflammation. Bacteriostatic test proves that it can suppress the growth of B-hemolytic streptococcus, staphylococcus aurous, diplococcus pneumonlae, meningococcus and colibacillus.

Manufacturer

China Wuhan Jianmin Pharmaceutical (Groups) Co. Ltd.

Wuhan Jianmin Pharmaceutical Factory

No. 384 Ying Wu Ave.

Hanyang, Wuhan, China

分析：《健民咽喉片说明书》原译共三段，没有结构语。第一段介绍药品的适用症、有效率和批准机构，第二段介绍药品成分和药物作用，第三段交代药品功能以及无副作用，最后是厂家名称和地址。根据药品说明书结构规范，改译增添了五个结构语："Composition""Actions & Indications""Adverse Reactions""Clinical Pharmacology"和"Manufacturer"，并对原译的结构和内容进行相应调整，便于海外读者定位所需信息。

[例2]　《急支糖浆说明书》英译体现样式调整

ACUTE BRONCHITIS SYRUP

Composition

Herba Houttuyniae cordata Thumb

Fagopyrum cymosum

Ilicis purpureae Hassk

Herba Ephedrae

Radix Asteris

Radix Peucedami

Fructus auranti

Radix Glycyrrhizae and adjuvants: Sucrose, Benzoic acid, Potassium sorbate.

Actions and Indications

Clearing heat and transform phlegm; diffuse the lung and suppress cough. Use for the treatment due to the external contraction of wind and fever with symptoms of an aversion to cold with fever, fullness and oppression in the chest and diaphragm, cough and sore pharynx; acute bronchitis, and acute attack of chronic bronchitis with the above mentioned symptoms.

Dosage and Administration

Adults	20 – 30 mL a time, 3 or 4 times a day, taken orally
Children ages 7 and older	15 mL a time, 3 or 4 times a day, taken orally
Children ages 3 to 7 years	10 mL a time, 3 or 4 times a day, taken orally
Children ages 1 to 3 years	7 mL a time, 3 or 4 times a day, taken orally
Children under 1 year	5 mL a time, 3 or 4 times a day, taken orally

Warnings

Do not use if you

—have allergic constitution.

Be cautious if you

—are taking tonic Chinese medicine or other drugs.

—are an athlete.

Ask a doctor for guidance before use if you

—are children, pregnant or breast-feeding women or an elderly.

—have hypertension, heart disease, diabetes and other chronic diseases such as liver disease and kidney disease.

Stop using and go to hospital

—if you have fever and body temperature more than 38.5℃, or has shortness of breath, or cough worsens with the amount of sputum increasing significantly.

—if the symptoms are not relieved after taking medicine for 3 days.

—if you have bronchiectasis, pulmonary abscess, pulmonale or tuberculosis, and show the symptom of cough.

Keep out of reach of children

Pharmacological actions

If the drug may interact with other drugs, ask your doctor or pharmacist for details.

Adverse drug reaction

No study report available.

Contraindication

No study report available.

Caution

Carefully read the Directions of Use.

Storage

Keep tightly close.

Package

Packaged in plastic bottle, 300 mL / bottle / box.

分析：借鉴说明书平行文本的排版形式对《急支糖浆说明书》进行格式调整，如逐行列出"Composition"中的药品成分，改用表格呈现"Dosage and Administration"具体内容，运用简洁明了的语言分行列出"Warning"具体条目等等。需要说明的是，当前对《急支糖浆说明书》的改译只限于排版上，原译存在的语言表达、语法等方面的问题将在下文阐述。

[例3] 《健民咽喉片说明书》功效语部分英译语言表达调整

原译：JIAN MIN YAN HOU PIAN is based on Xuan Mai Gan Jie Decoction, a proved formula from traditional Chinese medicine. It can clear pharynx, moisten throat to promote the production of body fluid, detoxify and purge the fire, and is effective for the temporary relief of acute and chronic pharyngitis symptoms.

对比句：润肺化痰、止咳平喘、护喉利咽、生津补气、调心降火。本品适用于伤风咳嗽、痰稠、痰多气喘、咽喉干痒及声音嘶哑。(《京都念慈菴蜜炼川贝枇杷膏说明书》)

对比句英译：Nin Jiom Pei Pa Koa is formulated from Chinese herbal ingredients and plant extracts together with honey and sugar syrups and has a pleasant taste. It provides temporary relief of coughs and sore throat associated with common cold, influenza or similar ailments. Nin Jiom Pei Pa Koa is effective for the temporary relief of the symptoms of bronchial cough and loss of voice.

改译：JIAN MIN YAN HOU PIAN is formulated from <u>Chinese herbal ingredients and plant extracts together with honey and sugar syrups</u> and has <u>a pleasant taste.</u> It can clear pharynx, moisten throat to promote the production of body fluid, detoxify and purge the fire, and is effective for the temporary relief of acute and chronic pharyngitis symptoms.

分析：《健民咽喉片说明书》首句说明药品基于中医药配方"玄麦甘桔汤"，对比文本《京都念慈菴蜜炼川贝枇杷膏说明书》首句，不仅突出其中草药和植物配方特点，还增加评价语"pleasant",给人以愉悦之感。译者可借鉴对比句具有感染力的表现手法,对《健民咽喉片说明书》译文进行调整,首先将抽象的产品成分介绍"a proved formula from traditional Chinese medicine"具体化,满足海外消费者对产品信息的需求;其次,增译"pleasant",给消费者直接的感受,增强产品吸引力。

第三节 段落的翻译

中成药说明书功效语部分是中成药说明书的重要组成部分,其主要功能是告知潜在消费者药品的药理功能和主治病症,这是药品的核心关键信息,也是海外消费者最看重的部分,将成为他们选择与购买药品最重要的依据(肖琼,2014:100)。规范的中成药英文说明书功效语翻译既要忠实体现原文原意,又要考虑海外受众接受度,通过准确、凝练的译文,精确传递信息,指导海外消费者用药。连贯与衔接问题是导致国外消费者难以理解功效语部分的重要原因,译者需要明确汉英在连贯与衔接方式上的不同,才能避免中式思维导致的结构不清的问题。

一、段落的对比分析

[**例1**] ① 止咳平喘。② 用于伤风感冒,鼻塞,流涕,咳嗽,气喘,痰多。(《咳喘丸说明书》)

原译:① This product relieve a cough, and smooth asthma, ② which used for people who catch a cold, have a stuffy nose, have a running nose, cough, gasping, and sputum.

对比句:① 精选天然草本植物精华,清热利咽,润喉护嗓。② 本品适合因长期用嗓、用声过度或因烟酒过多、睡眠不足所致的喉咙不适人士服用。(《清嗓饮说明书》)

对比句译文:① Voice Soothing Drink contains the natural herbal ingredients that help to expel heat, relieve sore throats, soothe and protect the voice. ② It is suitable for people who are suffering from sore throat due to excessive or prolonged use of their voice, excessive smoking and alcohol consumption or lack of sleep.

分析:《咳喘丸说明书》原译有明显的语法和语言表达问题。此外,药品功能和适应症是功效语两项同等重要的内容,但该译文中的主从句体现的是以药品功能为主,以药品适用症为辅的关系,逻辑关系表达不当。对比句译文连贯、衔接紧密、表达简洁,其中第①句交代产品的成分与功能,第②句说明适用对象及病症。

[例2] ① 清热化痰,宣肺止咳。② 用于外感风热所致的咳嗽,症见发热、恶寒、胸膈满闷、咳嗽咽痛;急性支气管炎、慢性支气管炎急性发作见上述证候者。(《急支糖浆说明书》)

原译:① Clearing heat and transform phlegm; diffuse the lung and suppress cough. ② Use for the treatment due to the external contraction of wind and fever with symptoms of an aversion to cold with fever, fullness and oppression in the chest and diaphragm, cough and sore pharynx; acute bronchitis, and acute attack of chronic bronchitis with the above mentioned symptoms.

对比句:① 和解少阳。② 本品适用于外感风寒或感冒后期所属少阳证。如寒热往来、食欲不振、头晕、作呕作闷、口苦咽干等症。(《小柴胡汤说明书》)

对比句译文:① Regulates Shaoyang disease. ② It is beneficial for relief of symptoms associated with Shaoyang disease due to the late stages of cold and flu such as chill and fever, loss of appetite, dizziness, nausea, bitter taste of mouth and dry throat.

分析:《急支糖浆说明书》原译采取直译的方法,除语言"硬伤"外,中式思维严重,连贯性与衔接性差。对比句译文第①句表明药品的功能,第②句表明适应证,体现了英语的语篇结构连接词多、衔接紧密的特色,通过"associated with""due to""such as"等词语显化语句之间的逻辑关系,内容重点突出,语言表达较为地道,易于海外消费者接受。

二、段落翻译的特点和策略

[例3] ① 止咳平喘。② 用于伤风感冒,鼻塞,流涕,咳嗽,气喘,痰多。(《咳喘丸说明书》)

改译:① This product functions to relieve cough and smooth breathing. ② It is suitable for people who are suffering from common cold, stuffy or running nose, cough, short breath and profuse sputum.

分析:以对比句为参考,调整《咳喘丸说明书》的翻译如下:(1)改变原译句型,突出药品功能和适应证两个信息重点,改译后的第①句介绍药品功能,第②句借用对比句中的"It is suitable for people who are"结构,说明药品的适用对象与适用症;

（2）为提升译文的结构平行度和语言简洁性,用"suffer from"词组改译适用对象与适用症部分;（3）调整译文中不符合原意的中医药术语英译,如"平喘"中的"喘"和西医中的"asthma"不是同一概念,改译为"short breath"。

[**例4**]　① 清热化痰,宣肺止咳。② 用于外感风热所致的咳嗽,症见发热、恶寒、胸膈满闷、咳嗽咽痛;急性支气管炎、慢性支气管炎急性发作见上述证候者。(《急支糖浆说明书》)

改译：① Acute Bronchitis Syrup can clear heat and transform phlegm, diffuse the lung and suppress cough. ② It is indicated for the relief of symptoms associated with cough due to external contraction of wind and fever, such as aversion to cold with fever, fullness and oppression in the chest and diaphragm, cough and sore pharynx, and for acute bronchitis and acute attack of chronic bronchitis with the same symptoms.

分析：对《急支糖浆说明书》原译进行调整如下：（1）基于对第②句各成分之间逻辑关系的分析,借用"be indicated for"和"symptoms associated with ... due to ... such as"句型对原译进行改译;（2）原译中两个句子分别是动名词和动词短语,为提升功效语译文的正式度,将原两个短语扩展为两个完整句。改译后,译文还存在中医药术语翻译的问题,将在词语部分进行深入分析和进一步调整。

第四节　词语的翻译

中成药药品名称承载着中医药文化和医理意义,好的药品译名应该既能传播中医药文化,又能激发海外消费者购买欲望。功效语部分的中医药专业术语蕴含着丰富的中医与中药学理论,用语偏文学化,介于文言文和白话文之间,含有大量的四字结构,是功效语英译的重点和难点。在翻译药品名称和中医药术语时,译者需要用海外消费者易于理解的表达方式,体现术语蕴含的中医药文化与医理特色。

一、词语的对比分析

1. 药品名称

[**例1**]　蛇胆川贝枇杷膏 SHEDAN CHUANBEI PIPA GAO

对比药名：念慈菴枇杷膏 Nin Jiom Pei Pa Koa（Traditional Chinese Herbal Cough

Syrup）

分析：根据 2006 年《中成药非处方药说明书规范细则》，药品名称必须标明与药典一致的通用名称和汉语拼音。李照国教授（2011：113 – 115）也认为，中药名称的翻译必须采取汉语拼音的形式，拉丁语和英文只能作为辅助说明。由于对于以英文为母语的西方读者而言，拼音词本身传达的意义有限（魏迺杰，1996：26 – 30），非常有必要在汉语拼音的后面加上剂型的英语名称，或加以必要的阐释。《念慈菴枇杷膏说明书》药品名称采取汉语拼音加注释的形式，方便海外受众了解该药品的属性、剂型及适用症。

［例 2］　余仁生猴枣化痰散 Children's Cough Powder

对比药名：同仁牛黄清心丸 Tongren Niuhuang Qingxin Wan（Cow-bezoar Sedative Bolus）

分析：《余仁生猴枣化痰散说明书》将药名译为"Children's Cough Powder"，虽然药品功能与适用症一目了然，但完全失去了中医内涵，不利于向海外传播中医文化。同仁堂的王牌产品"同仁牛黄清心丸"的药名英译包括汉语拼音和阐释两部分，表明了药品的成分、功效和剂型。

2. 功效语中的术语

功效语中的中医药术语存在误译、省译、欠额翻译等现象。为实现促进药品海外销售和推动中医药文化对外传播的双重目的，译者可以采取异化译法，保留、推广中医药术语约定俗成的译法，对于难以理解的中医药核心概念与表达，要用海外消费者能够理解的语言进行必要的解释与阐述。四字格是中医用语的一种非常重要的形式，是功效语术语翻译的重点和难点。尽管从表面上看，大部分中医四字术语由并列的两个二字词组构成，但它们彼此的语义关系并不像表面结构那么简单，各词素之间存在着一定的逻辑关系，这种关系完全由术语内涵决定。因此，确定术语格素之间的深层语义关系对中医术语翻译尤为重要（郑玲，2013：70 – 74）。

［例 3］　用于外感风寒，内伤湿滞，头痛昏重，脘腹胀痛，呕吐泄泻，胃肠型感冒。（《藿香正气胶囊说明书》）

原译：Cold induced fever; headaches and dizziness. Gastric pain and vomiting.

对比句：解表化湿，理气和中。适应症包括外感风寒，内伤湿滞，头痛，呕逆，胸满腹胀，伤暑，偶发性腹泻。（《藿香正气散颗粒说明书》）

对比句译文：Induce sweating to get rid of dampness, strengthen vital energy to regulate the stomach. For temporary relief of headache, common cold, indigestion, vomiting, abdominal distention, sunstroke and non-persistent diarrhea.

分析：《藿香正气胶囊说明书》译文省译了原文重要的概念与表达,中医文化内涵与医理几乎毫无体现。就其译文本身而言,逻辑关系不明,标点符号混乱,可读性较差。对比句介绍的是同样的药品的功效,但译文质量高出很多。对功能语中的中医文化负载词汇尽可能地进行意义阐释,保留了中医文化内涵与医理特征,表达简洁,重点突出,可作为原文的参考译文。

[**例4**] 清热化痰,宣肺止咳。用于外感风热所致的咳嗽,症见发热、恶寒、胸膈满闷、咳嗽咽痛;急性支气管炎、慢性支气管炎急性发作见上述证候者。(《急支糖浆说明书》)

原译：Acute Bronchitis Syrup can clear heat and transform phlegm, diffuse the lung and suppress cough. It is indicated for the relief of symptoms associated with cough due to external contraction of wind and fever, such as aversion to cold with fever, fullness and oppression in the chest and diaphragm, cough and sore pharynx, and for acute bronchitis and acute attack of chronic bronchitis with the same symptoms.

对比句1：扶助正气、祛病强身、温阳散寒、益气健脾。适用于体力衰弱、脾胃虚寒、咳嗽痰多、病后失调、机能退化及心脾两虚,气血不足所致的神疲体倦、食欲减退等症。(《养阴丸说明书》)

对比句1译文：Consolidate constitution and enhance health, warm yang, dissipate cold, reinforce qi and strengthen the spleen. Suitable for weakness in physical strength, tiredness, weakness and coldness in the spleen and stomach, cough with profuse sputum, imbalance of body after illness, deterioration of organs' function and for symptoms like tiredness, loss of appetite due to deficiency of the heart, the spleen, qi and blood.

对比句2：辛凉解表,清热解毒。适用于温病初起,风热感冒,发热,恶寒,鼻咽干热,咳嗽咽痛。(《银翘散颗粒说明书》)

对比句2译文：Induce sweating, clear away heat and eliminate toxic substances. For temporary relief of common cold with fever, cough and sore throat.

分析：《急支糖浆说明书》功效语原译存在中医术语翻译不准确的问题,如"外感风热"的"热"不能理解为"fever",应该是"heat"。此外还有欠额翻译的问题。由于缺乏对术语的充分解释,译文没有达到理想的沟通效果,海外受众很难理解术语的内涵,造成虽译又不译的状态。如"宣肺"译为"diffuse the lung",如不加以解释,没有中医药知识背景的海外消费者很难理解这个术语的意思。

对比句 1 出现了很多中医术语,译者一方面保留了约定俗成的术语表达,如"温阳"直接译为"warm yang","益气"译为"reinforce qi"。"yang"与"qi"在西方接受度较高,保留音译有益于传播中医药文化。同时,译者对不太重要或不太常见的中医术语,采用西方消费者熟悉的西医词汇或简洁易懂的语言进行解释,从而增强译语的可读性。如"扶助正气"和"祛病强身"意思相近,合并译为"consolidate constitution and enhance health","脾胃虚寒"译为"weakness and coldness in the spleen and stomach"。这样翻译虽然不能原汁原味地传递中医药内涵,但在保留中医术语核心意思的前提下,用西方受众易于理解的语言能够传递较好的交际意图。对比句 2 较完整地译出了药品的功能,保留了中医药文化与医理内涵,省译了西方受众难以理解且对全文意思影响不大的"温病"概念,并用简洁的介词短语突出主要适用症,译文流畅,重点突出,易于西方消费者理解。

二、词语翻译的特点和策略

[**例 5**] 蛇胆川贝枇杷膏

改译:蛇胆川贝枇杷膏 SHEDAN CHUANBEI PIPA GAO(Traditional Chinese Herbal Cough Syrup)

分析:借鉴《念慈菴枇杷膏说明书》药品名称英译采取的汉语拼音加注释的形式,"蛇胆川贝枇杷膏"药名改译采取了同样的方法。该方剂名称中含有两个以上的中药名,如果将方剂名称译出来比较长,会影响交际效果。因此,该类方剂名称一般采取音译。同时,后面进行了注释,便于海外受众了解该药品的属性、剂型及适用症。

[**例 6**] 余仁生猴枣化痰散

改译:余仁生猴枣化痰散 Yurensheng Houzao Huatan San(Rhesus Monkey Bezoar Powder for Children's Cough)

分析:借鉴同仁堂的王牌产品"同仁牛黄清心丸"药名英译方法,改译"余仁生猴枣化痰散",将其品牌名"余仁生"嵌入汉语拼音中,并在注释中交代药品主要成分、适用对象和适用症。

[**例 7**] 清热化痰,宣肺止咳。用于外感风热所致的咳嗽,症见发热、恶寒、胸膈满闷、咳嗽咽痛;急性支气管炎、慢性支气管炎急性发作见上述证候者。(《急支糖浆说明书》)

改译 1:Acute Bronchitis Syrup can clear heat to resolve phlegm, ventilate the lung qi to relieve cough. It is indicated for the relief of symptoms associated with cough due to external contraction of <u>wind and heat</u>, such as <u>fever</u>, <u>chill</u>, <u>distension over chest</u>, <u>cough</u>, <u>sore throat</u>, and also for acute bronchitis and acute attack of chronic bronchitis with the same symptoms.

改译2: Acute Bronchitis Syrup can <u>clear heat to resolve phlegm, ventilate the lung qi to relieve cough</u>. It is indicated for the relief of symptoms associated with cough, such as <u>fever, chill, chest distension and sore throat</u>, and also for acute bronchitis and acute attack of chronic bronchitis with the same symptoms.

分析: 借鉴例4给出的对比句1,对《急支糖浆说明书》功效语英译再作修改:(1)为更好地体现动词之间的逻辑关系,将"清热化痰""宣肺止咳"两个四字词语中动词的关系由并列改为目的;(2)采纳已有约定俗成、易于海外消费者理解的术语英语表达,如"咽痛"译为"sore throat","化痰"译为"resolve phlegm","宣肺止咳"译为"ventilate the lung qi to relieve cough"。对于英语中可以找到对应词的词语,如"恶风"的内涵与"chill"意思相近,可直接借用;(3)简化较为冗长的译文,如"胸膈满闷"原译文为"fullness and oppression in the chest and diaphragm",其中"满""闷"意思接近,可简化为"distension";"胸""膈"意思接近,可简译为"chest"。

改译1仍有不足之处,表现在术语较多、重点不突出,可能会影响海外受众对说明书中核心信息和中医药内涵的理解与吸收,因此可以进一步修改,通过适当省译与编译,用简洁易懂的语言传递最大的信息量。在改译1的基础上,参考例4给出的对比句2,对《急支糖浆说明书》的功效语再次改译,省译了理论较为深奥、西方受众难以理解的"外感风热",同时对适用症部分进行语法结构转换和语言浓缩,突出内容重点。

第五节　翻译练习与任务

一、翻译练习

1. 以下是广慈堂(Guang Ci Tang)"安神补心片(丸)"产品概述以及第一部分"WHAT DOES IT DO"内容①,分析其中的中医药术语(见画线部分)翻译方法、策略

---

① 来源: https://www.activeherb.com/anshen

以及交际效果。

An Shen Bu Xin Pian (An Shen Bu Xin Wan, SpiritCalm™, 安神补心片) is an all-natural Chinese herbal supplement that may calm the Heart and Spirit and support a peaceful mind and a restful sleep.

WHAT DOES IT DO

An Shen Bu Xin Wan is a common Chinese herbal remedy used to calm the mind and support a restful sleep.

From the perspective of Traditional Chinese Medicine (TCM), An Shen Bu Xin Wan calms the Heart and spirit and restores normal sleep rhythm by nourishing Heart Yin and blood while anchoring hyperactive Liver Yang (caused by deficient Heart blood). When blood is insufficient and therefore fails to nourish the Shen (spirit) which is said to be housed in the heart, a feeling of your heart pounding and having a trouble in falling asleep are common symptoms. An Shen Bu Xin Wan may also be used for mood swings and lightheadedness.

An Shen Bu Xin Wan is composed of 10 medicinal Chinese herbs that nourish Yin and blood, calm the Shen (spirit), clear heat and anchor Yang.

Dan Shen (Salvia root) regulates blood circulation, calms the Shen and dispels heat from the Heart. Dan Shen also nourishes blood to help heart beating. Studies have shown Dan Shen to have a marked calming effect. Shou Wu Teng (Fo-ti stem), also known as Ye Jiao Teng, nourishes the Heart and calms the Shen due to general blood deficiency while also clearing the meridian pathways.

Di Huang (Rehmannia root) is a powerful Yin tonic used to nourish the blood of the Heart.

Wu Wei Zi (Schisandra fruit) calms the heart and Shen, resolves anxiousness and dream-disturbed sleeplessness (which are signs of Yin and blood failing to nourish the heart). Tu Si Zi (Cuscuta seed) tonifies Kidney Yin and Yang and is combined with Wu Wei Zi to reduce the occurrence of frequent dreaming. Nu Zhen Zi (Glossy Privet fruit) clears heat caused by Yin deficiency and is a relatively mild tonic useful for lightheadedness. When combined with Wu Wei Zi, it is very useful for night sweats. Mo Han Lian, also known as Han Lian Cao (Eclipta) nourishes Yin and clears heat from the blood. It is often paired with Nu Zhen Zi for Liver and Kidney Yin deficiency.

Shi Chang Pu (Acorus) opens the orifices and calms the Shen. Zhen Zhu Mu (Mother of pearl) calms the Liver and anchors Yang, which can become hyper-ascendant due to Liver blood deficiency. Zhen Zhu Mu also clears Heart fire when combined with Shi Chang Pu.

He Huan Pi (Albizia Bark) calms the Shen and relieves Liver Qi stagnation (constraint).

2. 将以下句子译成英文①。

(1) 本品为最新滋补药。根据中医临床验方,采用丹参、朱砂、五味子等多味道地药材,以科学方法制成。

(2) "华佗再造丸"对脑血管意外所引起的出血性中风及脑血栓所引起的缺血性中风具有双向性的治疗作用,既可止出血,又可通血脉。

(3) 信宁咳可有效治疗由感冒或上呼吸道感染引起的咳嗽、急性和慢性支气管炎、哮喘性咳嗽、婴儿咳嗽等。

(4) 成人:初服1~2克(2~4片),以后每隔4小时服1~1.5克(2~3片)。

儿童:可根据年龄将成人剂量减少至1/2或1/4,或遵医嘱。

(5) 较少病人有胃肠道不适、头痛、血压降低或皮肤过敏反应等现象发生,不需特别处理,会逐渐消失。

二、翻译任务

对比分析汉英对照《云南白药胶囊说明书》,原译文存在误译、不简洁、标点符号误用、排版不醒目等问题。以小组的形式对原译进行改译,思考翻译过程中在语篇、段落、句子及词语层面所做的翻译调整、采取的翻译策略及原因。

云南白药胶囊说明书

请仔细阅读说明书并在医师指导下使用

本品含草乌(制);孕妇忌用;过敏体质及有用药过敏史的患者应慎用;外用前务必清洁创面

[**药品名称**]通用名称:云南白药

汉语拼音:Yunnan Baiyao Jiaonang

[**成　　分**]国家保密方,本品含草乌(制),其余成分略。

---

① 选自:李传英,潘承礼.医学英语写作与翻译[M].武汉:武汉大学出版社,2014:183-221.

[性　　状] 本品为硬胶囊,内容物为灰黄色至浅棕黄色的粉末;具特异香气,味略感清凉,并有麻舌感,保险子为红色的球形或类球形水丸,剖面呈棕色或棕褐色;气微,味微苦。

[功能主治] 化瘀止血,活血止痛,解毒消肿,用于跌打损伤,瘀血肿痛,吐血、咳血、便血、痔血、崩漏下血,手术出血,疮疡肿毒及软组织挫伤,闭合性骨折,支气管扩张及肺结核咳血,溃疡病出血,以及皮肤感染性疾病。

[规　　格] 每粒装 0.25 g

[用法用量] 刀、枪、跌打诸伤,无论轻重,出血者用温开水送服;瘀血肿痛与未流血者用酒送服;妇科各症,用酒送服,但月经过多、红崩,用温水送服。毒疮初起,服0.25 g,另取药粉,用酒调匀,敷患处,如已化脓,只需内服。其他内出血各症均可内服。

口服,一次 0.25 g～0.5 g,一日 4 次(二至五岁按 1/4 剂量服用;六至十二岁按1/2 剂量服用)。凡遇较重的跌打损伤可先服保险子一粒,轻伤及其他症状不必服。

[不良反应]　上市后不良反应监测数据及文献报道显示,极少数患者用药后出现以下不良反应:

1. 消化系统:恶心、呕吐、腹痛、腹泻、胃不适。

2. 呼吸系统:呼吸困难、呼吸急促、咽喉不适。

3. 皮肤及附件:眼睑水肿、皮肤发红、全身奇痒、躯干及四肢等部位出现荨麻疹。

4. 此外有高热、寒战、头晕、头痛、心悸、心慌、胸闷以及伪膜性结肠炎、急性胃炎、月经紊乱、过敏性休克等不良反应个案报告。

[禁　　忌] 1. 孕妇忌用。2. 对本品过敏者忌用。3. 皮肤及黏膜破溃、化脓者禁外用。

[注意事项]

1. 用药期间及停药后一日内,忌食蚕豆、鱼类及酸冷食物。

2. 外用前务必清洁皮肤,且仅用于毒疮初起时。

3. 过敏体质及有用药过敏史的患者慎用。

4. 严格按药品说明书用法用量使用,不宜长时间、大面积使用。

临床上确需使用大剂量给药,一定要在药师的安全监控下应用。

5. 如果出现不良反应或疑似不良反应,应立即停用(若外用应彻底清洁用药部位),并视症状轻重给予适当治疗。

6. 运动员慎用。

7. 本品含草乌(制),请仔细阅读说明书并在医师指导下购买和使用。

8. 如正在使用其他药品,使用本品前咨询医师或药师。

9. 请将本品放在儿童不能接触的地方。

[**药理毒性**]

1. 止血:明显促进大鼠及家兔的血小板凝聚、增强血小板的活化率及血小板表面糖蛋白的表达,能缩短大鼠及家兔的血液凝血时间、伤口出血时间及凝血酶时间,对家兔动脉血管有明显的收缩作用。

2. 活血化瘀:抑制大鼠静脉血栓形成,缓解高分子右旋糖苷造成大鼠微循环障碍,降低大鼠全血黏度,改善血液的血流状态,加快小鼠耳廓微循环速度,有一定的对抗大鼠毛细血管急性血栓形成的作用,不会出现血管内异常凝血。

3. 抗炎:对佐剂、角叉菜胶、异性蛋白、化学致炎剂及棉球肉芽肿等致炎因子造成的动物炎症模型均有明显的对抗作用。

4. 愈伤:可明显促进小鼠碱性成纤维细胞因子(bFGF)和血管内皮生长因子(VEGF)的生成,以及可显著促进大鼠手术区 bFGF 的表达和肉芽组织的增生。bFGF 与 VEGF 可促进成纤维细胞与血管内皮细胞的生成,因此可以加速血管的生长及结缔组织增生,达到促进伤口愈合的作用。

[**贮　　藏**]密封,置干燥处。

[**包　　装**]铝塑铝热带包装,每板装胶囊 16 粒、保险子 1 粒。

[**有 效 期**]60 个月。

[**执行标准**]《中国药典》2015 年版一部

[**批准文号**]国药准字 Z53020799

[**生产公司**]公司名称:云南白药集团股份有限公司

生产地址:云南省昆明市呈贡新区云南白药集团股份有限公司

邮政编码:650500

电话号码:40010000538

传真号码:0871－66226685

注册地址:云南省昆明市呈贡新区云南白药街 3686 号

网　　　址:www. yunnanbaiyao. com. cn

Yunnan Baiyao Capsules Instruction Manual

Please read the instruction carefully and use it under the guidance of physician

It contains Aconiti Kusnezoffii Radix Cocta; it is contraindicated in pregnant women and individuals with an allergic reaction to Yunnan Baiyao; be sure to clean the wound surface before external use.

[Pharmaceutical Name] Yunnan Baiyao Capsules

[Ingredients] National Secret Formula. It contains AconitiKusnezoffii Radix Cocta, other ingredients are omitted.

[Description] This product is hard capsule and the content is powder from grayish yellow to light brownish yellow; it has a special aroma, slightly cool taste and numbness in the tongue. The insurance pills are red spherical or spheroid-like waterpill with a brown or tan profile, a slight odor and bitter taste.

[Function and Indication] Eliminating blood stasis and hemostatic, promoting blood flow and analgesic, detoxifying and subsiding swelling. It is used for treatment of traumatic injury, stagnated blood swelling and pain, spitting blood, hemoptysis, hemotochezia, hemorrhoidal bleeding, metrorrhagia and metrostasia, suppurative and pyogenic infections and soft tissue bruise, closed fracture, brochiectasis and hemoptysis of pulmonary tuberculosis, ulcerative bleeding and infective disease on skin.

[Administration and Dosage] As to wounds by knife, bullet or traumatic injury, no matter how severe they have been, the capsules are administrated with warm boiled water by the bleeding wounded; The wounded suffer from stagnant blood, swelling and pain and no bleeding wounded take the capsules with wine; For patients suffer from diseases of gynecopathy take capsules with wine, but for those suffer from menorrhagia, metrorrhagia take capsules with warm boiled water. For initial stage of venenous sore, patient administer a dosage of 0.25 g and take another portion of medicine powder to mix homogeneously with wine which is used to apply on infectious part; for suppurative sore, oral administration is needed only. For slight injury and other internal hemorrhage symptom, capsules can be administered orally.

Oral administration: 1 - 2 capsules each time, 4 times daily (for children: 2 to 5 years old take 1/4 of dosage; 6 to 12 years old take 1/2 of dosage). For sever traumatic injury, a pill of Insurance pill can be administered at first, as to slight injury no Insurance pill will be needed.

[Adverse reaction] Monitoring data and literature reports of adverse reactions after marketing showed that very few patients had the following adverse reactions after medication:

1. Gastro-intestinal system disorders: nausea, vomiting, abdominalgia, diarrhea, stomach discomfort.

2. Respiratory system disorders: dyspnea, tachypnea, throat discomfort.

3. Skin and appendages disorders: eyelid edema, skin redness, general intense itching, urticaria in the trunk and limbs and others.

4. In addition, high fever, chills, dizziness, headache, palpitations, chest tightness, pseudomembranous colitis, acute gastritis, menstrual disorders, anaphylactic shock and other adverse reactions were reported in a few cases.

[Contraindication] 1: It is contraindicated in pregnant women.

2: It is contraindicated in individuals with an allergic reaction to Yunnan Baiyao.

3: It is contraindicated in defective or purulent skin and mucous membrane.

[Precautions]

1. Avoid fava beans, fish and cold sour food during medication and within one day after drug withdrawal.

2. Be sure to clean the skin before external use and only when malignant ulcer begins.

3. Be careful with allergic constitution and a history of drug allergy.

4. Use strictly according to the usage and dosage of the drug instructions, not suitable for long time and large area. It must be applied under the monitoring of doctors if necessary to use large doses of this medicine in clinic.

5. To discontinue immediately if adverse reactions or suspected adverse reactions occur (thoroughly cleaning the site of medication if external use) and appropriate treatment should be gived according to the severity of symptoms.

6. Athletes should use carefully.

7. It contains AconitiKusnezoffii Radix Cocta, please carefully read instruction manual and purchase and use it under the guidance of the physician.

8. To consult doctors before using it if other drugs are being used.

9. Keep out of reach of children.

[Pharmacological & toxicological effects]

1. Hemostatic effects: Promoting the aggregation of platelet in rat and rabbit significantly, enhancing the activity percentage and expression of surface glycoprotin of platelets, shortening the coagulation time of wounds and prothrombin time in rates and rabbits, demonstrating significantly constriction of artery vessel strip of rabbit.

2. Effects of promoting blood flow to eliminate blood stasis: Inhibiting thromogensis in vein of rats, remitting disturbance of microcirculation induced by high molecular dextrose in rats and improving the situation of blood flow, accelerating blood flow in auricle microcirculation of rats.

3. Anti-inflammatory action: Demonstrating significant antigonizing effects to the inflammatory models in animals induced by inflammation genesis factors, such as adjuvant, agar, foreign protein, inflammatory genesis chemicals and granuloma formation around cotton pellet.

4. Healing wounds effects: Promiting the production of (bFGF) (blast fibrocyte growth factor) and vessel endothelium growth factor (VEGF) in rays significantly, promoting the expression of (bFGF) in the field of operation in rats and granulation tissue proliferation. bFGF and VEGF may promote the production of vascular endothelial cell and blast figrocyte thus acccelerating the growth of blood vessels and connective tissue proliferation to achieve the effect of healing wounds.

[Specification] Each capsule content 0. 25 g.

[Storage] Keep airtight in a dry place.

[Package] Sealed in Aluminium-plastic-Aluminum bolt, 16 capsules per plate, 1 insurance pill.

[Validity] 5 years.

[Execution standard] The first edition of Chinese pharmacopoeia in 2015.

[Approval document number] GYZ No. Z53020799.

[Producer]

Name: Yunnan Baiyao Group

Address: Yunnan Baiyao Croup Col, Ltd. , Chenggong New District, Kunming, Yunnan Province, China

Postal code: 650500

Phone number: 4001000538

Fax number: 0871－66226685

Registered address: Number 3686 in Baiyao Street, Chenggong District, Kunming City, Yunnan Province

Website: www. yunnanbaiyao. com. cn

三、扩展阅读

［1］李照国. 中医英语翻译教程［M］. 上海：上海三联书店,2019.

［2］李传英,潘承礼. 医学英语写作与翻译［M］. 武汉：武汉大学出版社,2014.

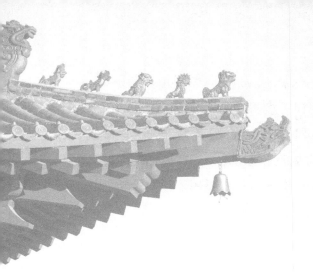

第七章
中医药企事业单位
网页简介英译

在"一带一路"倡议的时代背景下,我国中医药国际化进程逐步加快,推动了越来越多的中医药产品和服务产业跨出国门。中医药企事业单位奉行"走出去"的发展战略,积极扩大对外交流与合作,不断开拓中医药国际市场,稳步提高产品与服务的国际竞争力。2019年4月,商务部办公厅、国家中医药管理局办公室印发《关于开展中医药服务出口基地建设工作的通知》,提出建设一批以出口为导向、具有较强辐射带动作用的基地,形成一批中医药服务世界知名品牌。中医药企事业单位宣传资料是海外用户和消费者了解中医药企事业单位情况、主要产品及其服务项目的窗口。英文网页是向海外展示中国企事业单位形象的名片。中医药企事业单位通过英文网页宣传资料,力争为海外潜在顾客提供信息,增强产品与服务项目的吸引力,提升中医药国际影响力。

第一节 语 料 导 入

本节的分析语料分为两组。第一组为中文简介和原译,选自中国中医科学院广安门医院、中国北京同仁堂(集团)有限责任公司、天津天士力医疗健康投资有限公司、江苏省中医院、西安中医脑病医院、三亚市中医院、山东中医药大学等首批17家国家中医药服务出口基地的网页,以及中国医药保健品股份有限公司、广州医药集团有限公司、南京中医药大学等国内知名中医药公司、高校的网页。该组语料代表国内中医药企事业单位网上英文简介的平均水平。第二组为英文简介,选自哈佛医学院

（Harvard Medical School）、美国加州大学洛杉矶分校医疗中心（UCLA Health Care）、罗氏公司（Roche）、百时美施贵宝公司（Bristol-Myers Squibb）等国外知名医学院、医院和生物制药公司的网页，代表该文体的英文规范和标准。文中只对简介文字部分进行语料分析，而忽略图表等其他部分。本节列出的语料主要用于语篇分析，没有列出的段落和词语分析语料将在第三节和第四节分别呈现。

一、中文语料（包括原译）

1.《中国医药保健品股份有限公司简介》①

中国医药保健品股份有限公司是在上海证券交易所挂牌的国有控股上市公司（股票简称：中国医药；证券代码：600056），其控股股东为中央骨干公司中国通用技术（集团）控股有限公司。公司秉承"关爱生命、追求卓越"的核心理念，致力于医药产业发展和人类健康事业，努力打造中国医药领域的旗舰公司。

公司已经建立了以国际贸易为引领、以医药工业为支撑、以医药商业为纽带的科工贸一体化产业格局，产业形态涉及研发、种植加工、生产、分销、物流、进出口贸易、学术推广、技术服务等全产业链条。

在医药研发生产领域，公司拥有两家博士后科研工作站及一大批高素质研发专家，曾获国家科技进步二等奖；公司拥有国内领先的化学原料研发生产平台，国内先进的特色化学药、现代中药研发生产平台，在抗感染类、抗病毒类药物的研发生产以及甘草等药材及其制品的种植加工领域处于领先地位。

在国际贸易领域，作为医药行业进出口领域传统专业主渠道，公司始终保持着领先地位，且在政府项目业务领域具备传统实力和特色优势。天然药物贸易业务坚持全产业链专业化发展模式，有机整合天然药物种植、仓储、加工、销售等产业链环节，在行业内居于领先地位。医药化工贸易业务经营范围涵盖化学原料及制剂、生物及血液制品各品规、全领域，可为顾客提供一流的医药化工贸易集成服务。医疗器械贸易业务致力于为顾客提供全过程项目集成化服务，并与世界各著名医疗器械生产厂商建立了稳固的合作关系，在进口和分销领域处于国内领先地位。健康领域大宗商品业务涉及保健食品原料、大宗农产品、精细化工原材料等，在一些重点商品进出口贸易领域有较高知名度。

---

① 中文简介来源：通用技术中国医药官网，搜索日期：2013 - 03 - 12，转引自陈小慰（2017：170）。
英文简介来源：通用技术中国医药官网，搜索日期：2013 - 03 - 12，转引自陈小慰（2017：185）。

在国内医药商业领域,公司已逐步建立起以高端、特色产品为核心,具有产业价值链整合协同优势的医药商业体系,已形成以北京、广东、江西、河南、河北、湖北、新疆为重点,覆盖全国的营销网络体系,并在所在区域具有较高的知名度和品牌影响力。公司建有大型物流中心,具备完善的经营资质,可为广大合作伙伴提供全方位的增值服务。

面向未来,中国医药着力在重点产品领域建立横跨国内和国际两个市场的营销网络,聚焦现代中医、特色化学制剂和生物制药等核心产业领域,打造集研发、生产、销售、服务于一体的产业链,努力将公司发展成为一家在国内医药行业中具有重要地位、在国际市场具有较强竞争力和品牌影响力的科工贸一体化大型公司集团。

China Meheco Co., Ltd., is a state-holding company listed at Shanghai Stock Exchange (Ticker Symbol: China Meheco; Stock Code: 600056) and its controlling shareholder is China General Technology (Group) Holding Co., Ltd., an important backbone state-owned enterprise directly administered by the central government. Upholding the tenet of "Cherishing Life and Seeking Excellence", China Meheco is dedicated to the promotion of human health and the development of pharmaceutical industry, endeavoring to become a flagship pharmaceutical enterprise in China.

China Meheco has established a comprehensive business framework that is guided by international trade, supported by pharmaceutical manufacture and coordinated by pharmaceutical commerce. Its business scope fully covers the whole industry chain, from R&D, cultivation & processing, manufacturing, distribution, logistics to international trading, academic promotion and technical service, etc.

In the future, the company will focus on building sales network in both domestic and international markets for core products of modern Traditional Chinese Medicine, distinctive chemical preparation and bio-pharmaceutical preparations, to create an industrial chain which fully integrates R&D, production, sales and services. China Meheco strives to become a large-scale integrative pharmaceutical group with high position among domestic peers, and with worldwide renown for its great brand influence and high competitiveness.

China Meheco owns two post-doctoral workstations and a group of experts, including secondary prize winners of the National Prize for Progress in Science and Technology; it also owns a first-class platform in China for production and processing of

APIs, distinctive preparations and modern Traditional Chinese Medicines. The corporation takes lead in R&D and production of antibiotics and anti-virus products, and also in the cultivation and processing of licorice and other herbal products.

2.《山东中医药大学简介》①

山东中医药大学创建于 1958 年,1978 年被确定为全国重点建设的中医院校,1981 年成为山东省重点高校,是教育部本科教学工作水平评估优秀学校、山东省人民政府和国家中医药管理局共建中医药院校、山东省应用基础型人才培养特色名校、山东省首批高等学校协同创新中心、山东省首届省级文明校园、山东省一流学科建设单位、省属高校绩效考核优秀单位。

学校在省属高校中拥有国家级重点学科最多,首批获得硕士、博士学位授权,首批设立博士后科研流动站,首批成为国家“973”项目首席承担单位。硕士点数量位居全国同类院校前列。

学校紧紧围绕立德树人根本任务,坚持社会主义办学方向,全面贯彻党的教育方针,秉承“厚德怀仁、博学笃行”的校训,坚持“以文化人、厚重基础、注重传承、勇于创新”的办学特色,顽强拼搏、砥砺奋进,经过几代人辛勤耕耘和不懈奋斗,培养出十余万中医药人才和健康服务相关专业人才。

学校致力于高水平中医药大学建设,2007 年由济南市历下区主体迁入扁鹊故里——长清,现在学校三校区(含青岛中医药科学院)办学,总占地 2 000 余亩,建筑面积 53.9 万平方米。学校图书馆馆藏纸质图书 201 万册、电子图书 75.4 万册、古籍善本 3 万册,为山东省古籍重点保护单位。设置 17 个教学机构、5 个科研机构、4 个教辅机构,拥有 3 所直属附属医院、17 所非直属附属医院、24 所教学医院,10 家山东省研究生联合培养基地、18 家中医局住院医师规范化培训基地。有 1 个国家级实验教学示范中心、1 个国家级大学生校外实践教育基地。

学校坚持立德树人、大医精诚,努力培养高素质专门人才。拥有 28 个本科专业,涉及医、理、文、工、管、法、教育等学科门类;有中医学、中药学、中西医结合 3 个博士学位授权一级学科、15 个二级学科,9 个硕士学位授权一级学科、46 个硕士二级学科;拥有中医博士专业学位授予权和中医、中药学、药学、生物医学工程、护理学硕士专业学位授予权。截至目前,学校全日制在校生 21 000 余人,其中研究生 3 000 余人。学

---

① 中文简介来源: https://www.sdutcm.edu.cn/xxgk/xxjj.htm,搜索日期: 2020 - 02 - 01。
英文简介来源: https://www.sdutcm.edu.cn/xxgk/English/Homepage.htm,搜索日期: 2020 - 02 - 01。

校与 40 余所国外知名大学、医疗机构建立了长期友好合作关系。

学校坚持师德为先、教学为要,拥有实力雄厚的师资队伍。现有教职医护员工 3 400 余人,其中博士生导师 174 人,硕士生导师 683 人。荣获国家"国医大师"荣誉称号者 3 人,"全国名中医"3 人,"岐黄学者"3 人,"973"项目首席科学家 1 人,全国优秀教师 8 人,中医药高等学校教学名师 2 人,山东省教学名师 10 人,山东省优秀教师 6 人,山东省"泰山学者"特聘专家 10 人,山东省"泰山学者"攀登计划专家 1 人,省部级有突出贡献的中青年专家 26 人,享受国务院特殊津贴专家 52 人,山东省名中医药专家 96 人,"山东名老中医"6 人。有山东省优秀教学团队 6 个,山东省十大优秀创新团队 1 个,"全国高校黄大年式教师团队"1 个。荣获省级以上教学成果奖 58 项。

学校坚持突出特色、争创一流,形成一批优势和特色学科专业。现有中医基础理论、中医医史文献、中医内科学 3 个国家重点学科,中医学、中药学 2 个山东省一流学科,国家中医药管理局重点学科 29 个;国家临床重点专科 13 个,国家中医药管理局重点专科 21 个;有中医学、中药学、针灸推拿学和制药工程 4 个国家级特色专业,11 个省级特色专业;拥有 2 个山东省高水平应用型重点建设专业群、3 个重点培育专业群;3 个专业(群)获山东省教育服务新旧动能转换专业对接产业项目立项。建成 10 门在线开放课程上线运行。

学校坚持以文化人、以文育人,积极打造特色鲜明的文化品牌。学校充分发挥孔孟之乡、扁鹊故里、针灸发源地的文化优势,坚持把中医文化和齐鲁文化作为以文化人的重要资源,塑造独具特色的大学文化品格。成立了全国首家省级中医药文化协同创新中心;获批省内首家中医药智库——山东省中医药政策与管理研究基地。策划承办第八届世界儒学大会——儒家思想与中医药文化专题论坛,成立儒医文化研究会,首次将中医药文化推向高层次国际学术平台。成功立项国家中医药管理局国际合作专项——中国—波兰中医药中心,引领全省高校在"一带一路"建设上取得实质性突破。山东省中医药博物馆获批为全国中医药文化宣传教育基地、山东省中医药文化宣传教育基地、山东省中医药文化旅游示范基地、山东省第十一批社会科学普及教育基地。

学校培养的人才具有"敦厚朴实、基础扎实、工作踏实"的鲜明特点,涌现出一批获得"全国三好学生""中国大学生自强之星标兵""山东青年五四奖章"等荣誉称号的优秀学生,在第二届全国《黄帝内经》知识大赛总决赛中学校获得总冠军。在全国第四届"互联网+"创新创业大赛中,金银花新品种培育与种植技术推广项目获得大赛金奖,这是全国中医药院校自大赛举办以来首次获得金奖。

学校注重科技创新驱动,打造一流科研平台,取得丰硕成果。现有中医学、中药学、中西医结合3个博士后科研流动站,设有1个国家教育部重点实验室,6个国家中医药管理局三级重点实验室,2个国家中医药管理局重点研究室,2个全国学术流派传承工作室,33个全国名老中医药专家传承工作室,2个山东省重点实验室,4个山东省工程技术研究中心,1个山东省示范工程技术研究中心,1个山东省工程实验室,4个山东省高等学校协同创新中心,7个山东省高校科研创新平台。十二五以来,共承担厅局级以上科研课题686项,其中国家级项目198项,连续获得山东省科技进步一等奖8项。建校以来,获国家级和省部级一等奖奖励的科研成果共计29项,拥有国家中医临床研究基地、国家重大新药创制平台(山东)中药单元平台。

新时代谱写新篇章,新征程再创新辉煌。学校将坚持以习近平新时代中国特色社会主义思想为指导,贯彻落实全国教育大会精神,坚持全面从严治党,坚持立德树人根本任务,坚持以人民为中心发展思想,坚持推动学校内涵式发展,不忘初心、牢记使命,深化高等教育综合改革,提高人才培养质量,办好人民满意大学,努力在服务健康中国健康山东和新时代现代化强省征程中争创一流、走在前列,奋力谱写一流学科和高水平中医药大学高质量发展新篇章!

INTRODUCTION TO SHANDONG UNIVERSITY
OF TRADITIONAL CHINESE MEDICINE

Shandong University of Traditional Chinese Medicine (SDUTCM) was founded in 1958, listed as one of the key state construction TCM higher-learning institutes in 1978, and approved as one of the key Shandong provincial universities in 1981. It is currently the only independent medical university in Shandong Province, and rated excellent in the national undergraduate education evaluation conducted by the Ministry of Education. It is among the first batch of "five preeminent featured universities" approved by Shandong provincial government. Among all the colleges and universities in Shandong province, it takes the lead in the number of the state key disciplines, in offering master's and doctoral programs and post-doctoral research programs, and also in undertaking the state "973 Projects" as a chief organization.

SDUTCM adheres to the motto of "Cultivating virtues and harboring benevolence, learning extensively and practicing persistently", exploits fully the advantages of traditional Chinese medicine, strengthens its connotation construction, and as a result forms its own educational features, namely "nurturing students' minds by culture, consolidating their foundation, emphasizing knowledge inheritance, and encouraging innovation". It has trained tens of thousands graduates with professional skills for the nation and society. They share something distinctive in common, for instance, honest-and-sincere personality, solid professional basis, down-to-earth work attitudes. Some of them have won national honorary titles, such as "National Three-Goods Students", "Self-Reliance Star of Chinese University Students", and "May 4th Youth Medal of Shandong Province", etc.

SDUTCM has been striving for the goal of becoming one of preeminent featured universities. In 2007, the main campus moved from Lixia District, Jinan City, to Changqing District—the hometown of Bianque (a famous physician in ancient China), covering a total area of 122 hectares with a building area of 545,000 square meters. The facilities and equipment are valued at over RMB 192,765,000, and the library has a collection of 1,871,000 paper books, 509,000 electronic books and 30,000 rare ancient books. The library is a "Shandong provincial key protection unit of ancient books". It has 14 colleges, 3 directly-affiliated hospitals, 11 indirectly-affiliated hospitals, 24 teaching hospitals, 97 clinical teaching bases, 10 Shandong graduates jointly-training bases. It has one national experimental teaching demonstration center and one national undergraduate off-campus education and practice bases.

SDUTCM works hard to train high-quality talents and TCM physicians by both cultivating virtues and encouraging learning. It has 21 undergraduate programs, involving the fields of medicine, sciences, humanities, engineering and management. Meanwhile, it has 3 first-rate doctoral degree authorization disciplines, including traditional Chinese medicine, traditional Chinese materia medica and combination of TCM and western medicine, entitled to confer 15 doctoral degrees. It also offers 8 first-rate master's degree authorization disciplines, entitled to confer 44 master's degrees, which involve all the second-rate disciplines of traditional Chinese medicine, traditional Chinese materia medica and combination of TCM and western medicine, which have already started to permeate to peripheral disciplines. Additionally, SDUTCM has been authorized to grant doctoral degrees in clinical medicine and master's degrees in clinical medicine, traditional Chinese materia medica, pharmacy and biomedical engineering. At present, it has an enrollment of nearly 21, 000 students, including nearly 18, 000 undergraduates and over 2, 700 postgraduates. SDUTCM attaches great importance to international academic exchange and cooperation. It has built long-term cooperative relationships with over 30 prestigious foreign universities and medical organizations. It now has about 200 overseas Chinese and foreign students.

SDUTCM has a strong teaching faculty, with over 3, 900 staff members. Amongst them, there are 110 doctorate supervisors, 422 master supervisors, 2 "Great Master of National Medicine", 1 chief scientist of the State "973" Projects, 8 "National Outstanding Teachers", 10 "Outstanding Teacher of Shandong Province", 6 "Outstanding Teaching team of Shandong Province", one "Shandong Top Ten Excellent Innovation Team", 8 Shandong provincial "Taishan Fellowship" Professors, 20 "Young and Middle-aged Breakthrough-Contribution Experts" at provincial or ministerial level, 44 "State Council Special Allowance" recipients, 63 "Shandong Provincial Famous TCM Specialists".

SDUTCM has been focusing on its features construction and excellence, and has formed a batch of dominant and featured disciplines. It now owns 3 state key disciplines, namely Basic Theory of traditional Chinese Medicine, History and Literature of TCM and Traditional Chinese Internal Medicine, 29 State TCM Administration key disciplines, 14 provincial key disciplines, 23 state key specialist clinics, 19 provincial key specialist clinics, 4 state characteristic specialties, namely Traditional Chinese Medicine, Traditional Chinese Materia Medica, Acupuncture and Tuina, and Pharmaceutical Engineering, 1 Education Ministry key reform pilot specialty, 11 provincial characteristic specialties, 3 national high-quality open courses, and 33 provincial high-quality courses.

SDUTCM has forged numerous first-class scientific research platforms by introducing the sci-tech and innovation drive. It has 3 post-doctoral stations in the disciplines of traditional Chinese medicine, traditional Chinese materia medica and combination of TCM and western medicine, 1 Education Ministry key laboratory, 6 State TCM Administration level-3 key laboratories, 2 State TCM Administration key research centers, 2 Shandong provincial key laboratories, 3 Shandong provincial engineering technological research centers, 1 Shandong provincial engineering laboratory. It leads one collaborative innovation centre of Shandong provincial colleges and universities. Since the "National 11th Five-Year Plan" period, SDUTCM has undertaken 1093 scientific research projects at bureau level or above. Amongst them, there are 244 national projects. Since its founding, SDUTCM won 2 awards on the First National Scientific Conference, 3 state sci-tech advance second prizes, 3 state technical innovation awards, and 13 provincial sci-tech advance first prizes. SDUTCM has been recognized by the Ministry of Science and Technology as one of the "Technological Supporting Institutions for Promoting the Key Projects of State Sci-tech Achievements", and as one of the "Undertaking Institutions for the Projects of Modernized, Industrialized and Standardized Plantation of Chinese Materia Medica". SDUTCM has one national clinical research base, one national innovation platform of new drug on TCM unit, and one Shandong provincial research base of humanities and social sciences.

On the course of constructing a high-level distinctive TCM university, SDUTCM always upholds the socialism direction, bases on virtues cultivation, develops by innovation, and is oriented by economic growth and social progress. It centers on talents training, focuses on its core TCM disciplines, highlights TCM features, emphasizes cultural inheritance and innovation, strengthens connotation construction, and deepens educational reform, for the purpose of constantly improving talents training quality, comprehensively promoting educational strength, and nurturing qualified builders and reliable successors for Chinese characteristic socialism, with an integrated development in morality, intelligence, sports and arts.

3. 《西安中医脑病医院简介》①

西安中医脑病医院是陕西省中医药管理局批准和直管的三级甲等中医专科医院,开放床位800张,主要从事脑积水、脑瘫、智力低下、孤独症、癫痫、植物人、中风、脑外伤、脑肿瘤、渐冻人等脑病的治疗与康复。

承担国家中医诊疗重点研究室1个,国家中医学术流派传承工作室1个,国家级及省级重点学科3个,重点专科8个,牵头重点专科优势病种中医诊疗方案和临床路径4个、中医临床诊疗指南4个,获国家专利5项,主持、参与国家、省、市科研课题59项,研发中医诊疗设备3种,获省部级科技成果奖9项,出版专著5部。

医院是国家、省、市残联确定的残疾人康复人才培养基地,先后完成了各级残联

---

① 中英文简介来源:西安中医脑病医院官网,搜索日期:2021-06-01。

下达的肢体矫治手术、运动功能障碍、智力障碍、脑瘫、孤独症等残疾患者的康复训练任务。

近年来，在"一专两心三佳四型五位一体"发展战略引领下，秉承"德勤精诚，爱脑济民"的院训，内强素质，外塑形象，全面提升医疗服务质量，现已基本形成集医疗、教学、科研、文化、连锁为一体，以西安为中心，面向全国，辐射国外的医疗格局，努力把医院建设成规模适度、功能完善、环境优美、设施完备、管理规范、技术精湛的三级甲等示范中医专科医院。

三级甲等中医专科医院

国家儿科重点学科

国家儿科临床重点专科

国家中医脑病重点专科

国家十二五康复重点专科

国家中医药管理局脑性瘫痪中医诊疗重点研究室

国家中医药管理局西岐中医儿科学术流派传承工作室

国家中医药管理局基层中医药服务能力提升工程实施单位

国家中医药管理局区域诊疗中心培育项目(儿科、康复科)实施单位

国家中医药管理局重大疑难疾病(脑梗死)中西医临床协作单位

中残联、陕西省残联、西安市残联康复定点医院

中残联孤独症儿童康复教育试点项目机构

陕西省中医特色康复服务示范基地

陕西省"三秦学者"创新团队

陕西省"千人计划"创新项目实施单位

陕西省"百人计划"项目实施单位

石学敏院士专家工作站

马融儿童脑病工作室

刘华为名老中医传承工作室西安中医脑病医院工作站

陕西省名中医工作室

陕西省中医住院医师规范化培训基地协同单位(脑病学科、康复学科、儿科学)

陕西省残疾孤儿手术康复"明天计划"定点医院

陕西省残疾人康复中心脑瘫治疗中心、康复研究中心

陕西青年志愿者助残"阳光行动"服务基地

陕西省优生优育协会"摇篮工程"儿童脑损伤康复示范基地

西安中医脑病医院博士后创新基地

陕西中医药大学研究生培养基地

陕西中医药大学真实世界临床研究院脑病分院

西安交通大学生命科学与技术学院研究生实习基地

陕西省省级机关事业单位职工医保定点医院

陕西省、西安市新农合、城镇职工、居民、工伤、康复医保定点医院,跨省结算单位

Hospital Profile

Xi'an TCM Hospital of Encephalopathy is affiliated to Shaanxi University of Chinese Medicine, Xi'an Medical College and Shaanxi Energy Institute, make every effort to governance with medical treatment, teaching, scientific research and chain management, now has developed into one class-A hospital of traditional Chinese medicine, has 800 beds, mainly engaged in diagnosis and rehabilitation of cerebral palsy, mental retardation, autism, stroke, brain trauma, epilepsy, vegetative patients, hydrocephalus, brain tumors, ALS and other brain diseases. The hospital is the disabled rehabilitation talent training base of the national, provincial and municipal, undertaking surgical correction of all levels of disabled persons' federation, the assessment and rehabilitation work for patients with physical disabilities, mental retardation and mental disability.

Adhering to the motto of "Diligent and sincere, love brain and help people", the hospital continuously strengthens its quality and shapes its image externally. It not only devotes itself to studying assiduously for patients' healing, but also makes unremitting efforts to improve patients' humanized medical experience. The hospital strive to achieve the long-term development goals of medical care, education, scientific research, culture and chain operation. The hospital with a professional technology as the core competitiveness, the discipline and specialized subject construction characteristics of TCM, The hospital carries out chain operation in Shaanxi province, as well as Shanghai, Fujian, Xinjiang, Inner Mongolia and other provinces and cities, serving local patients, striving to achieve the goal of being based in Shaanxi, facing the whole country and going to the world.

In the past 20 years, the hospital has focused on academic exchanges and cooperation with foreign countries, and has received many visitors from more than 20 countries and regions including the United Kingdom, the United States, Portugal, Israel, France, Switzerland, Australia, Mongolia, Japan, India, Thailand, and Gambia. Experts and scholars came to our hospital for international medical exchanges on Chinese medicine and international consultations on difficult diseases. In response to the "One Belt One Road" initiative, has treatment more than 12,000 patients from Russia, Bangladesh, Ukraine, Kazakhstan, Tajikistan, Kyrgyzstan, Uzbekistan and other etc. of more than 10 countries and regions along "One Belt One Road", successively established the Chinese Characteristic Medical Care (Bangladesh) Center, the World Federation of Acupuncture Chinese Traditional Medical Care (Indonesia) Center, Huatuo Traditional Medical Care (Indonesia) Center, the Tibetan Medicine (Ufa) Cooperation Center of the Republic of Bashkorstan, Russia, Kazakhstan Nursultan BI-Zhuldyzai Rehabilitation International Medical Association and Xi'an International Cerebral Palsy Rehabilitation Center in Kazakhstan, sent a number of medical teams to foreign countries for international medical exchanges, various forms of international exchanges and cooperation in traditional Chinese medicine, and the spread of traditional Chinese medicine culture and diagnosis and treatment characteristics technology.

Grade-A tertiary specialized hospital of TCM

National key subject project construction unit on TCM paediatrics

National clinic key specialty project construction unit on TCM paediatrics

National key specialty project construction unit on TCM encephalopathy

The Twelve fifth national key specialty project construction unit on rehab

National cerebral palsy TCM treatment research laboratory construction unit

National Xiqi paediatrics TCM academic school heritage work room construction unit

National basic level Chinese medicine service capacity improvement project implementation unit

National regional diagnosis and treatment center cultivation project (pediatrics, rehabilitation) implementation unit

National Clinical Cooperation Unit of Chinese and Western Medicine for major difficult and complicated diseases (Cerebral Infarction)

China Disabled Persons' Federation autistic children rehabilitation education pilot project organization

Graduate Training Base of Shaanxi University of Chinese Medicine

Graduate Training Base of Xi'an Medical College

Graduate Practice Base of Life Science and Technology college of Xi'an Jiaotong University

Encephalopathy Branch of Real World Clinical Research Institute of Shaanxi University of Chinese Medicine

Chairman and Secretary-General unit of Specialty Committee of Cerebral Palsy of the World Federation of Chinese Medicine Societies

二、英文语料

1. Get to Know Roche in Brief(《罗氏公司简介》)①

A pioneer in healthcare

We have been committed to improving lives since the company was founded in 1896 in Basel Switzerland. Today, Roche creates innovative medicines and diagnostic tests that help millions of patients globally.

The frontrunner in personalised healthcare

Roche was one of the first companies to bring targeted treatments to patients. With our combined strength in pharmaceuticals and diagnostics, we are better equipped than any other company to further drive personalised healthcare. Two-thirds of our Research and Development projects are being developed with companion diagnostics.

The world's largest biotech company

We are the world's number 1 in biotech with 17 biopharmaceuticals on the market. Over half of the compounds in our product pipeline are biopharmaceuticals, enabling us to deliver better-targeted therapies.

The global leader in cancer treatments

We have been at the forefront of cancer research and treatment for over 50 years, with medicines for breast, skin, colon, ovarian, lung and numerous other cancers.

The leading provider of in vitro diagnostics

We offer doctors profound information to guide treatments and to answer more

---

① 来源：https://www.rochecanada.com/about,搜索日期：2020-07-30。

patients' questions than any other company. And our tests enable hospitals and labs to deliver that information quickly and reliably.

A committed investor in innovation

We invest around 9 billion Swiss francs in Research and Development every year because innovation is our lifeblood. This is amongst the highest Research and Development spends in the world across all industries.

An extraordinary workplace

We are a force of over 90,000 people working together across more than 100 countries. Roche is consistently ranked as employer of choice by its employees and by external institutions.

A sustainable company

For many years running we have been recognized by the Dow Jones Sustainability Indices as the leader in sustainability within our industry.

2. About Harvard Medical School(《哈佛医学院简介》)①

Since the School was established in 1782, faculty members have improved human health by innovating in their roles as physicians, mentors and scholars. They've piloted educational models, developed new curricula to address emerging needs in health care, and produced thousands of leaders and compassionate caregivers who are shaping the fields of science and medicine throughout the world with their expertise and passion.

Our Mission

To nurture a diverse, inclusive community dedicated to alleviating suffering and improving health and well-being for all through excellence in teaching and learning, discovery and scholarship, and service and leadership.

Members of the Harvard Medical School community have also excelled in the research arena. Faculty members have been making paradigm-shifting discoveries and achieving "firsts" since 1799, when HMS Professor Benjamin Waterhouse introduced the smallpox vaccine to the United States. Their accomplishments are recognized internationally, and, in fact, 15 researchers have shared in nine Nobel prizes for work

---

① 来源: https://hms.harvard.edu/about-hms, 搜索日期: 2020 - 07 - 30。

completed while at the School.

The Faculty of Medicine includes more than 11, 000 individuals working to advance the boundaries of knowledge in labs, classrooms and clinics. The School's main quadrangle in Boston houses nearly 200 tenured and tenure-track faculty members in basic and social science departments as well as in classrooms where students spend their first two years of medical school.

But teaching and research extend beyond the Quad. Harvard Medical School has affiliation agreements with 15 of the world's most prestigious hospitals and research institutes, vital partners that provide clinical care and training. They also serve as home base for more than 10, 000 physicians and scientists with faculty appointments.

With its vast reservoir of talent, extensive network of affiliates and commitment to problem solving, Harvard Medical School is uniquely positioned to steer education and research in directions that will benefit local, national and global communities.

The History of HMS (Omitted)

Campus and Culture (Omitted)

Facts and Numbers (Omitted)

HMS Affiliates (Omitted)

LCME Accreditation (Omitted)

Social Media Hub (Omitted)

Leadership (Omitted)

Contact HMS (Omitted)

Transforming the Future of Human Health (Omitted)

3. About Us: Best Healthcare, Latest Medical Technology(《加州大学洛杉矶分校医疗中心简介》)①

UCLA Health is among the most comprehensive and advanced health care systems in the world. Together, UCLA Health and the David Geffen School of Medicine at UCLA strive every day to be a model that redefines the standard of excellence in health care. It is our integrated mission to provide state-of-the-art patient care, to train top medical professionals and to support pioneering research and discovery.

---

① 来源：https://www.uclahealth.org/about-us,搜索日期：2020 - 07 - 30。

UCLA Health is comprised of:

Ronald Reagan UCLA Medical Center

UCLA Medical Center, Santa Monica

UCLA Mattel Children's Hospital

Stewart and Lynda Resnick Neuropsychiatric Hospital at UCLA

UCLA Health Clinics

UCLA Faculty Group

David Geffen School of Medicine at UCLA

Our physicians are world leaders in the diagnosis and treatment of complex illnesses, and our hospitals are consistently ranked among the best in the nation by U. S. News & World Report.

Research achievements

UCLA Health is at the cutting edge of biomedical research, and our doctors and scientists are pioneering work across an astounding range of disciplines, from organ transplantation and cardiac surgery to neurosurgery and cancer treatment, and bringing the latest discoveries to virtually every field of medicine.

Facts about UCLA Health

More than 200 UCLA physicians are listed among the Best Doctors in America

Nearly 600,000 unique patients per year

2. 5 million outpatient clinic visits

80,000 Emergency Department visits

40,000 hospital stays

3,300 total faculty

2,700 clinical faculty

600 basic science faculty

1,200 residents and fellows

4,000 registered nurses

20,000 employees

Service available

And as an academic medical center, we are able to offer our patients the latest technologies as well as access to potentially life-saving new therapies and leading-edge clinical trials. With a comprehensive array of research and clinical centers, addressing topics from stem cell biology, AIDS, gene therapy, neurosciences, women's health and geriatrics, UCLA continues to define what an academic medical center can be. UCLA Health's commitment to patient care, research and education means that our patients benefit from the latest diagnostic and treatment techniques in virtually every area of medicine.

Community service

And we are a committed community partner. In fact, more than 70 percent of our medical students and some 200 faculty participate in community health programs each year. Some of those programs include training Los Angeles firefighters and paramedics to treat stroke victims on-site; and addressing a multitude of child health and welfare issues at the Center for Healthier Children, Families and Communities.

第二节 篇章的翻译

汉英简介在体裁结构、主要内容和文体正式度方面差异明显,为实现译文的信息和感染功能,从语篇宏观层面对原文进行调整显得尤为重要,对于质量差和不符合目的语文化与行文习惯的原文,在译前很有必要进行修改(刘季春,2016:228-231)。

一、篇章的对比分析

1. 纲要式结构

汉英网上简介平行文本在语篇内容和结构上普遍存在差异。下面分别以医药公司、医学院校和医院简介为例进行对比分析。

1)《中国医药保健品股份有限公司简介》和"Get to Know Roche in Brief"(《罗氏公司简介》)纲要式结构对比分析

《中国医药保健品股份有限公司简介》没有小标题,全文较为平淡,信息重点不够突出。首段介绍了行业定位、核心理念和发展目标,中间部分重点介绍公司经营产品与服务范围,以及研发与创新信息,最后交代公司发展前景。相比较而言,罗氏公司简介的语篇结构更清晰,信息重点更突出。简介的 8 个小标题 "A pioneer in healthcare"（医疗保健的先驱者）、"The frontrunner in personalised healthcare"（个性化医疗保健领域的领先者）、"The world's largest biotech company"（世界上最大的生物技术公司）、"The global leader in cancer treatment"（癌症治疗的全球领导者）、"The leading provider of in vitro diagnostics"（体外诊断的领先提供者）、"A committed investor in innovation"（致力于创新的投资者）、"An extraordinary workplace"（不同寻常的工作场所）和"A sustainable company"（持续发展的公司）凸显了集团定位和亮点，突出体现了"公司能够为消费者提供什么样不同一般的产品及服务"（陈小慰，2017：175），直观、鲜明地树立了一个在个性化医疗服务、癌症治疗、体外诊断等领域处于领先地位，致力于不断创新、可持续性发展，值得消费者信任的医疗行业先驱者形象。

2）《山东中医药大学简介》和"About Harvard Medical School"（《哈佛医学院简介》）纲要式结构对比分析

《山东中医药大学简介》首段宏观介绍了学校的性质、定位与荣誉，中间部分采取平铺直叙的方法，详尽介绍了学校的历史溯源、地理位置及占地面积、学科门类与专业及学位点、学生情况、师资水平、科研水平、重点实验室与基地建设情况、获奖情况、国际交流与合作、学校发展目标，最后全文以标语口号式的套语结束。可以说，该简介突出体现了注重整体性的中文修辞传统，全文面面俱到，信息高度密集，力图全方位展示高校的整体形象。哈佛医学院简介的正文部分高度概括了哈佛医学院的卓越贡献，然后重点介绍了学校在教育、科研、医疗服务方面的使命，并在正文后提供了 9 个链接，分别是"The History of HMS"（哈佛医学院历史）、"Campus and Culture"（校园与文化）、"Facts and Numbers"（事实与数字）、"HMS Affiliates"（哈佛医学院成员）、"LCME Accreditation"（LCME 专业认证）、"Social Media Hub"（社会媒体中心）、"Leadership"（领导力）、"Contact HMS"（联系哈佛医学院）和"Transforming the Future of Human Health"（改变人类健康未来），每个链接又引出新的信息，感兴趣的读者可以点击以获取所需信息。例如读者点开"Facts and Numbers"小标题链接，可以看到有关学科门类、专业及学位、学生情况、师资水平、科研情况等事实与数字，这些信息以数据条目的形式列出，一目了然。

3）《西安中医脑病医院简介》和"About Us：Best Healthcare，Latest Medical Technology"（《加州大学洛杉矶分校医疗中心简介》）纲要式结构对比分析

《西安中医脑病医院简介》篇幅较短，第一段概述医院定位及治疗的主要脑病类型，第二段列举科研实力，第三段突出该院是残疾人康复人才培养基地，第四段详述发展战略、院训和发展格局，最后罗列医院的 30 多个资质、工作室和示范基地头衔。

《西安中医脑病医院简介》英语版在中文简介的基础上对语篇内容和结构进行了调整。第一段全面介绍医院在脑病和残疾人康复方面的医疗服务特色,第二段介绍其使命和院训,第三段介绍医院海外合作和交流活动情况,译文最后部分选择性地列出国家级别的医院资质、工作室和示范基地头衔。可以说,《西安中医脑病医院简介》英译考虑到海外受众信息需求,在语篇内容和结构上进行了合理的调整。

加州大学洛杉矶分校医疗中心简介的结构清晰,在引言段介绍了中心的医疗服务在全球的卓越地位和中心使命,正文介绍了该医疗体系的构成,并分别从研究成就(Research achievements)、关于 UCLA 医疗中心的事实(Facts about UCLA Health)、提供服务(Service available)、社会服务(Community service)四个方面进行详述。在"提供服务"部分,通过描述各种服务,令读者的亲切感和参与感油然而生,体现了英文简介注重"我能为您提供什么"的理念。

2. 体现样式

汉语简介的作者和读者心理距离较远,往往用词较为正式,公文体特点明显,而英语简介的作者和读者心理距离较近,通常采用非正式的日常语复现语域,用词亲切。下面分别以《中国医药保健品股份有限公司简介》和《山东中医药大学简介》部分段落为例,对比分析汉英文本在体现样式方面的差异。

[例1]　① 中国医药保健品股份有限公司是在上海证券交易所挂牌的国有控股上市公司(股票简称:中国医药;证券代码:600056),其控股股东为中央骨干公司中国通用技术(集团)控股有限公司。② 公司秉承"关爱生命、追求卓越"的核心理念,致力于医药产业发展和人类健康事业,努力打造中国医药领域的旗舰公司。

原译:① China Meheco Co., Ltd., is a state-holding company listed at Shanghai Stock Exchange (Ticker Symbol: China Meheco; Stock Code: 600056) and its controlling shareholder is China General Technology (Group) Holding Co., Ltd., an important backbone state-owned enterprise directly administered by the central government. ② Upholding the tenet of "Cherishing Life and Seeking Excellence", China Meheco is dedicated to the promotion of human health and the development of pharmaceutical industry, endeavoring to become a flagship pharmaceutical enterprise in China.

对比句:① We have been committed to improving lives since the company was founded in 1896 in Basel Switzerland. ② Today, Roche creates innovative medicines and diagnostic tests that help millions of patients globally.

分析:该段为《中国医药保健品股份有限公司简介》首段,原译第①句以公司国有背景开头,强调其国有特点,第②句陈述公司的理念和使命。该段采用第三人称,诉诸国家和政府权威,使译文看上去像官方文件,与受众的直接关联不足,不容易引发海外受众的兴趣。对比句选自《罗氏公司简介》,第①句以"we"为主语,交代公司使命及成立时间和地点,第②句概述公司的成就和贡献。对比句采取消费者视角,语气显得亲切随和,以为顾客具体提供怎样的全面服务打动受众。

[**例2**] ① 学校紧紧围绕立德树人根本任务,坚持社会主义办学方向,全面贯彻党的教育方针,② 秉承"厚德怀仁、博学笃行"的校训,③ 坚持"以文化人、厚重基础、注重传承、勇于创新"的办学特色,④ 顽强拼搏、砥砺奋进,⑤ 经过几代人辛勤耕耘和不懈奋斗,培养出十余万中医药人才和健康服务相关专业人才。

原译:② SDUTCM adheres to the motto of "Cultivating virtues and harboring benevolence, learning extensively and practicing persistently",(增译)exploits fully the advantages of traditional Chinese medicine, strengthens its connotation construction, ③ and as a result forms its own educational features, namely "nurturing student' minds by culture, consolidating their foundation, emphasizing knowledge inheritance, and encouraging innovation". ⑤ It has trained tens of thousands graduates with professional skills for the nation and society.

对比句:① As global citizens, we work sustainably, responsibly and seek to give back. ② Through the Bristol-Myers Squibb Foundation, we promote health equity and strive to improve health outcomes of populations disproportionately affected by serious diseases and conditions, giving new hope to some of the world's most vulnerable people.

分析:该段原文介绍山东中医药大学的办学理念、校训和办学特色,通过运用四字词语增强修辞效果。原译选择性译出原文中实质性信息,省译了西方读者难以了解或无须了解的第①句,并增译了"exploits fully the advantages of traditional Chinese medicine, strengthens its connotation construction",以体现学校的中医药特色。译文用词正式,引号部分的校训和办学特色译文略显冗长。英文平行文本选自百时美施贵宝公司官网简介,首句简明扼要地介绍了公司的理念与发展目标,第②句用长句展开阐述。"seek to""give new hope to""sustainably""responsibly"等词简明易懂、生动形象,增强了译文的感染力和吸引力。

二、篇章翻译的特点和策略

鉴于汉英网上简介的语篇内容和结构差异,按照中文简介进行全文逐字翻译显然不合适。为了实现译文预期交际效果,译者应围绕西方受众的信息需求,重视实质信息和事实表述,突出受众想了解的信息。对于西方受众可能觉得乏味无用的内容、空洞的评论信息,或程式化用语,需要简化或省略。在结构调整方面,应按照西方受众的阅读习惯,先主后次,正文重点介绍学校定位、性质、使命、价值观等重点内容,细节以小标题或链接形式列在后面,相关的事实和数据宜集中在专栏列出。

[例3] 《西安中医脑病医院简介》翻译调整

Xi'an TCM Hospital of Encephalopathy

We are a Class-A tertiary TCM hospital integrating treatment, training, research, culture and chain operation with a commitment to improving your brain health with our virtues, diligence, persistence and sincerity. To improve the overall medical service level and construct a positive hospital image, we have basically built a Xi'an-based medical pattern facing the nation and aiming overseas.

1. Services available

We are comprehensively improving the quality of medical services, so that you can experience the perfect functions, beautiful environment, complete facilities and exquisite technology of our hospital.

We are mainly engaged in diagnosis and rehabilitation of cerebral palsy, mental retardation, autism, stroke, brain trauma, epilepsy, vegetative patients, hydrocephalus, brain tumors, ALS and other brain diseases. As the municipal, provincial and national training base for the rehabilitation of the disabled, the hospital can help you with the rehabilitation training tasks such as limb correction surgery, dyskinesia, mental retardation, cerebral palsy and autism.

2. International exchange & cooperation

The hospital focuses on academic exchanges and cooperation with more than 20 countries and regions. In the past 20 years, the hospital has:

—received experts and scholars for international medical exchanges on TCM and international consultations on difficult diseases;

—treated more than 12000 patients from more than 10 countries and regions along the Belt and Road;

—successively established the medical care center overseas, including TCM Medical Care (Bangladesh) Center, the World Federation of Acupuncture TCM Care (Indonesia)

Center, Huatuo TCM Care (Indonesia) Center, the Tibetan Medicine (Ufa) Cooperation Center of the Republic of Bashkorstan, Russia, Kazakhstan Nursultan BI-Zhuldyzai Rehabilitation International Medical Association and Xi'an International Cerebral Palsy Rehabilitation Center in Kazakhstan;

—sent a number of medical teams to foreign countries for international medical exchanges, international exchanges and cooperation in TCM, and the spread of TCM culture, diagnosis and treatment technology with TCM characteristics.

3. Facts & numbers

Research achievements:

—1 national key research laboratory of TCM diagnosis and treatment

—1 national academic school inheritance studio of TCM

—3 national and provincial key disciplines

—8 key specialties

—4 TCM diagnosis and treatment programs and clinical pathways for dominant diseases in key specialties

—4 TCM clinical diagnosis and treatment guidelines

—5 national patents

—59 national, provincial and municipal scientific research projects

—3 kinds of TCM diagnosis and treatment equipment

—9 provincial and ministerial scientific and technological achievement awards

—5 monographs

Honors:

—Class-A tertiary specialized hospital of TCM

—National key subject project construction unit on TCM paediatrics

—National clinic key specialty project construction unit on TCM paediatrics

—National key specialty project construction unit on TCM encephalopathy

—The Twelve fifth national key specialty project construction unit on rehab

—National cerebral palsy TCM treatment research laboratory construction unit

—National Xiqi paediatrics TCM academic school heritage work room construction unit

—National basic level Chinese medicine service capacity improvement project implementation unit

—National regional diagnosis and treatment center cultivation project (pediatrics, rehabilitation) implementation unit

—National Clinical Cooperation Unit of Chinese and Western Medicine for major difficult and complicated diseases (Cerebral Infarction)

—China Disabled Persons' Federation autistic children rehabilitation education pilot project organization

—Graduate Training Base of Shaanxi University of Chinese Medicine

—Graduate Training Base of Xi'an Medical College

—Graduate Practice Base of Life Science and Technology college of Xi'an Jiaotong University

—Encephalopathy Branch of Real World Clinical Research Institute of Shaanxi University of Chinese Medicine

—Chairman and Secretary-General unit of Specialty Committee of Cerebral Palsy of the World Federation of Chinese Medicine Societies

分析：为了更加符合目标受众的信息需求和阅读习惯，借鉴对比文本对《西安中医脑病医院简介》进行改译。调整后的译文首先介绍医院定位、理念和使命，正文分为三个部分，并配以标题，第一部分"Services available"介绍医院在脑病治疗和残疾人康复方面的特色，第二部分"International exchange & cooperation"分项列出医院的国外交流和合作活动，第三部分"Facts & numbers"分别列出医院科研特色、成就和重要荣誉。为提升译文的亲切度和外观醒目度，改译适当运用第一人称和第二人称，并重新排版。需要说明的是，翻译调整主要针对原译的语篇结构，译文可能仍存在语言、拼写、表达等方面的问题。

[例4]　①中国医药保健品股份有限公司是在上海证券交易所挂牌的国有控股上市公司（股票简称：中国医药；证券代码：600056），其控股股东为中央骨干公司中国通用技术（集团）控股有限公司。②公司秉承"关爱生命、追求卓越"的核心理念，致力于医药产业发展和人类健康事业，努力打造中国医药领域的旗舰公司。

改译：② Caring for life and aiming to make the best even better, we are a pharmaceutical specialist in China dedicated to the promotion of human health and the development of pharmaceutical industry. ① As a state-holding company listed at Shanghai Stock Exchange (Ticker Symbol: China Meheco; Stock Code: 600056),

169

China Meheco Co., Ltd. is strongly supported by its controlling shareholder, China General Technology (Group) Holding Co., Ltd., a leading state-owned enterprise directly administered by the central government. ①

分析:陈小慰(2017:184-185)采用第一人称对《中国医药保健品股份有限公司简介》进行改译,体现了英文简介以用户和消费者为中心的理念。译文按照英文公司简介规范,首先交代公司的理念和使命,第②句再介绍其国有特点。

[**例5**] ① 学校紧紧围绕立德树人根本任务,坚持社会主义办学方向,全面贯彻党的教育方针,② 秉承"厚德怀仁、博学笃行"的校训,③ 坚持"以文化人、厚重基础、注重传承、勇于创新"的办学特色,④ 顽强拼搏、砥砺奋进,⑤ 经过几代人辛勤耕耘和不懈奋斗,培养出十余万中医药人才和健康服务相关专业人才。

改译:(增译)As a TCM-specialized university, ② we adhere to the motto of cultivating students with virtues, benevolence, knowledge and practice. ③ Our education, as a result, forms the feature of nurturing minds with Chinese culture, encouraging innovation while emphasizing TCM knowledge inheritance. ④⑤ After years of persistent effort, we have produced more than 100,000 TCM talents and health service-related professionals.

分析:在对《山东中医药大学简介》进行段落翻译调整时,借鉴英语平行文本简洁易懂的语言特色,对原译的长句进行简化处理,将引号中的四字词语改用通俗的语言表达,最后一句强调培养的是"TCM talents and health service-related professionals",呼应上文提出的学校办学理念。

第三节 段落的翻译

一、段落的对比分析

1. 内容和结构

完成语篇层面的内容和结构调整后,还需按照英文简介规范对每段内容和结构进行相应调整。现以《江苏省中医院简介》为例予以说明。

---

① 来源:陈小慰.译有所依——汉英对比与翻译研究新路径[M].厦门:厦门大学出版社,2017:70.

[例1]　① 江苏省中医院(南京中医药大学附属医院)创建于 1954 年 10 月,为全国首批成立的省级中医医院之一,② 首任院长叶橘泉为中科院学部委员。③ 建院 60 多年来,经过几代人的励精图治,辛苦耕耘,坚持以中医为本,突出中医药特色优势,国医大师、名医群体荟萃。①

原译：① Yuxiu Zhongshan, Longpan Tiger, Jinling Ancient Capital, and Jiangsu Provincial Hospital of Traditional Chinese Medicine (Affiliated Hospital of Nanjing University of Traditional Chinese Medicine) near Xinjiekou have now passed the glorious year of Jiazi. In October 1954, with the care of the Party and the government, the cradle of New Chinese Medicine was born, which brought together the famous doctors of the Yangtze and Huaihe River, the descendants of imperial doctors and the descendants of Menghe and Wumen medical schools. ② Ye Juquan, a well-known Chinese medicine physician and member of the Academy of Chinese Sciences, was the first president. (增译) Tan Zhenlin, then President of Jiangsu Provincial People's Government, issued a letter of appointment for the president. (增译) Mr. Guo Moruo wrote the name of Jiangsu Traditional Chinese Medicine Hospital in his own hand. ②

对比句：① UCLA Health is among the most comprehensive and advanced health care systems in the world. ② Together, UCLA Health and the David Geffen School of Medicine at UCLA strive every day to be a model that redefines the standard of excellence in health care. ③ It is our integrated mission to provide state-of-the-art patient care, to train top medical professionals and to support pioneering research and discovery. ③

分析：与《江苏省中医院简介》汉语简介相比,英译首句增加了许多信息,如医院的历史渊源、地理位置,成立时汇集江淮名医、御医后代和孟河、吴门医派传人,以及文化负载词"jiazi";第②句和中文简介一致,介绍首任院长叶橘泉,随后增译时任江苏省人民政府主席谭震林颁发院长任命书,以及郭沫若给医院题字等信息。译文添加的内容导致该段内容琐碎,重点信息不突出。对比文本《加州大学洛杉矶分校医疗中心简介》开篇聚焦定位和使命,简短明确,可使受众一下抓到信息要点,其中第①句开门见山,指出该中心是世界上最全面、最先进的医疗体系之一,第②句说明中心的努力目标,第③句具体指出医院使命。

---

① 来源：http://www.jshtcm.com/list.php?fid=66,搜索日期：2020 - 02 - 01。
② 来源：http://en.jshtcm.com/us/#/about,搜索日期：2020 - 02 - 01。
③ 来源：https://www.uclahealth.org/about-us,搜索日期：2020 - 07 - 30。

2. 连贯与衔接

[**例 2**] ① 学校是世界卫生组织(WHO)传统医学合作中心、国际针灸培训中心,② 是教育部批准接收和培养外国留学生及港澳台地区学生的首批高等中医药院校之一,已经为五大洲培养留学生 3 万余名。③ 1993 年学校与澳大利亚皇家墨尔本理工大学(RMIT)合作开办中医学专业,首开我国与西方正规大学合作开展中医学历教育先河。④ 2010 年 6 月 20 日,时任国家副主席习近平出席了我校与 RMIT 合作建立的中医孔子学院揭牌仪式并发表重要讲话,对我校办学水平给予高度评价。⑤ 在教育部的支持下,2019 年 2 月学校又与爱尔兰国立大学(高威)签约共建中医与再生医学孔子学院,该孔子学院的建立是贯彻落实习近平总书记"用开放包容的心态促进传统医学和现代医学更好融合",推进中医药新时代海外发展的积极探索。⑥ 学校已经与 90 多个国家和地区的高等院校或学术团体及机构有着广泛交流和合作,先后在大洋洲、欧洲、美洲建立了 8 个海外中医药中心。①

原译: ① The university is WHO Collaborating Center for Traditional Medicine designated by the World Health Organization, and is International Acupuncture Training Center approved by the Ministry of Health, ② and is one of the first advanced Chinese Medicine institutions authorized by the Ministry of Education to enroll international students as well as students from Taiwan, Hong Kong and Macao. ③ In 1993, NJUCM pioneered the practice of cooperating with RMIT University, Australia to facilitate the Bachelor program of Chinese Medicine. (增译) NJUCM makes every effort to promote the understanding of Chinese Medicine in foreign countries with special focus in developing Confucius Institute and overseas Chinese Medicine Center. ④ A leading Chinese Medicine Confucius Institute was established by NJUCM in collaboration with RMIT University, Australia on June 20, 2010. Mr. Xi Jinping attended the opening ceremony and delivered keynote speech. ⑥ NJUCM currently has extensive communication and contact with over 90 countries and regions worldwide, and has established partnership with higher education institutions, government agencies and academic groups in over 30 countries and regions. It has established 8 overseas Chinese Medicine Centers in succession respectively in Oceania, Europe and America. Its three TCM centers, Sino-Australia, Sino-Switzerland and Sino-France centers have become national-level overseas

---

① 来源: http://www.njucm.edu.cn/2014/0722/c285a4242/page.htm,搜索日期: 2021 - 06 - 01。

Chinese medicine center. ①

分析：该段谈论的是南京中医药大学（NJUCM）为促进国际学术交流而做的五项大事，原译遗漏了原文第⑤句，但在译文第③句和第④句间增译一句，概述该中心在海外建立孔子学院和中医海外中心方面作出的不懈努力。译文只有一段，平铺直叙，不易读者抓住每项事件的主要内容。

[**例3**]　① 学校坚持师德为先、人才引领，拥有实力雄厚的师资队伍。② 现有教职医护员工3 500余人，③ 其中博士生导师176人，硕士生导师828人。④ 荣获国家"国医大师"荣誉称号者3人，"全国名中医"3人，"岐黄学者"2人，"973"项目首席科学家1人，全国优秀教师8人，中医药高等学校教学名师2人，山东省教学名师10人，山东省优秀教师7人，山东省"泰山学者"特聘专家10人，山东省"泰山学者"攀登计划专家1人，省部级有突出贡献的中青年专家27人，享受国务院特殊津贴专家52人，山东省名中医药专家94人，"山东名老中医"6人。有山东省优秀教学团队6个，山东省十大优秀创新团队1个，"全国高校黄大年式教师团队"1个。连续两届获国家教学成果二等奖，荣获省级以上教学成果奖58项。②

原译：①② SDUTCM has a strong teaching faculty, with over 3,900 staff members. ③④ Amongst them, there are 110 doctorate supervisors, 422 master supervisors, 2 "Great Master of National Medicine", 1 chief scientist of the State "973" Projects, 8 "National Outstanding Teachers", 10 "Outstanding Teacher of Shandong Province", 6 "Outstanding Teaching team of Shandong Province", one "Shandong Top Ten Excellent Innovation Team", 8 Shandong provincial "Taishan Fellowship" Professors, 20 "Young and Middle-aged Breakthrough-Contribution Experts" at provincial or ministerial level, 44 "State Council Special Allowance" recipients, 63 "Shandong Provincial Famous TCM Specialists". ③

分析：《山东中医药大学简介》的正文段落平铺直叙各种资源、荣誉成就，或使用大量的数据，导致篇幅冗长，信息重点不突出，读者也无法快速找到所需数字和事实。对比之下，英文简介常常用"Facts & Numbers"将数据和事实用专栏列出，使得文本更贴近海外受众的思维习惯，在阅读的第一时间就能够获取直观数据。

---

① 　来源：http://english. njucm. edu. cn/295/303/，搜索日期：2021－06－01。

② 　来源：https://www. sdutcm. edu. cn/xxgk/xxjj. htm，搜索日期：2020－02－01。

③ 　来源：https://www. sdutcm. edu. cn/xxgk/English/Homepage. htm，搜索日期：2020－02－01。

二、段落翻译的特点和策略

汉英简介具有不同的连贯和衔接特点,如果进行直译,译文会显得结构臃肿、条理不清。这种情况下可对译文进行重组,简化臃肿的段落,明晰逻辑关系,这样易于读者提取主要信息。举例说明如下。

1. 内容和结构

[**例4**] ① 江苏省中医院(南京中医药大学附属医院)创建于 1954 年 10 月,为全国首批成立的省级中医医院之一,② 首任院长叶橘泉为中科院学部委员。③ 建院 60 多年来,经过几代人的励精图治,辛苦耕耘,坚持以中医为本,突出中医药特色优势,国医大师、名医群体荟萃。

改译: ① Established in October 1954, Jiangsu Hospital of Traditional Chinese Medicine is one of the first provincial hospitals of TCM in China. ② Ye Juquan, a well-known Chinese medicine physician and member of the Academy of Chinese Sciences, was the first president. ③ Over the past 60 years, the hospital has attracted renowned TCM masters and doctors from all over the country, and improved human health by adhering to TCM as the basis, and by highlighting TCM features.

分析: 改译后的《江苏省中医院简介》首段第①句简要介绍医院定位和成立时间,第②句介绍首任院长,第③句介绍医院特色和成就。江淮名医、御医后代和孟河、吴门医派传人等细节,以及谭震林和郭沫若等历史背景信息可移至正文后面的栏目专门介绍。

2. 连贯与衔接

[**例5**] ① 学校是世界卫生组织(WHO)传统医学合作中心、国际针灸培训中心,② 是教育部批准接收和培养外国留学生及台港澳地区学生的首批高等中医药院校之一,已经为五大洲培养留学生 3 万余名。③ 1993 年学校与澳大利亚皇家墨尔本理工大学(RMIT)合作开办中医学专业,首开我国与西方正规大学合作开展中医学历教育先河。④ 2010 年 6 月 20 日,时任国家副主席习近平出席了我校与 RMIT 合作建立的中医孔子学院揭牌仪式并发表重要讲话,对我校办学水平给予高度评价。⑤ 在教育部的支持下,2019 年 2 月学校又与爱尔兰国立大学(高威)签约共建中医与再生医学孔子学院,该孔子学院的建立是贯彻落实习近平总书记"用开放包容的心态促进传统医学和现代医学更好融合",推进中医药新时代海外发展的积极探索。⑥ 学校已经与 90 多个国家和地区的高等院校或学术团体及机构有着广泛交流和合作,先后

在大洋洲、欧洲、美洲建立了8个海外中医药中心。

改译：① As the WHO Collaborating Center for Traditional Medicine designated by the World Health Organization, and the International Acupuncture Training Center, NJUCM has:

② —become one of the first batch of Chinese medicine universities approved by the Ministry of education to enroll international students and students from Taiwan, Hong Kong and Macao, and has trained more than 30,000 foreign students form five continents;

③ —initiated the Bachelor program of Chinese Medicine together with Royal Melbourne Institute of Technology (RMIT) in 1993, pioneering TCM academic education program in cooperation with Western regular universities;

④ —held the opening ceremony of the Confucius School of Chinese medicine established by NJUCM in association with RMIT in June, 2010, during which Vice President Xi Jinping delivered a keynote speech;

⑤ —signed a contract with the National University of Ireland (Galway) to build the Confucius Institute of TCM and regenerative medicine to integrate the traditional medicine with modern medicine;

⑥ —established exchanges and cooperation with higher education institutions or academic groups in over 90 countries and regions, and set up 8 overseas TCM centers in Oceania, Europe and America up till now.

分析：改译根据英文简介表达习惯，在总起段增译"NJUCM has"统领下文，并用"become""initiated""held""signed""established"等动词开头，分项、分行列出每个事件，信息突出，一目了然。

[例6]　① 学校坚持师德为先、人才引领，拥有实力雄厚的师资队伍。② 现有教职医护员工3 500余人，③ 其中博士生导师176人，硕士生导师828人。④ 荣获国家"国医大师"荣誉称号者3人，"全国名中医"3人，"岐黄学者"2人，"973"项目首席科学家1人，全国优秀教师8人，中医药高等学校教学名师2人，山东省教学名师10人，山东省优秀教师7人，山东省"泰山学者"特聘专家10人，山东省"泰山学者"攀登计划专家1人，省部级有突出贡献的中青年专家27人，享受国务院特殊津贴专家52人，山东省名中医药专家94人，"山东名老中医"6人。有山东省优秀教学团队6个，山东省十大优秀创新团队1个，"全国高校黄大年式教师团队"1个。连续两届获国家教学成果二等奖，荣获省级以上教学成果奖58项。

改译：① We possess strong teaching staff, focusing on the morality construction of teachers and the leading role of professionals.

Facts & Numbers: ②③④

—Total faculty: 3,500

—Doctorate supervisors: 176

—Master supervisors: 828

—Great Master of National Medicine: 3

—Chief scientist of the State 973 Projects: 1

—National Outstanding Teachers: 8

—State Council Special Allowance recipients: 52

分析：改译根据英文简介规约，在正文中只保留概述性的第①句话，而将本段②③④句有关数字归拢到"Facts & Numbers"栏目，根据数字类型进行分类。此外，英文简介注重国际和国家权威机构颁发的奖项，因此改译只保留国家级有代表性的称号和奖项。

[例7] ① 以同仁堂国药集团在香港建立生产基地为标志，② 实现了从"北京的同仁堂"向"中国的同仁堂""世界的同仁堂"跨越，③目前已经在五大洲 28 个国家和地区设立经营服务终端，④ 加快了中医药国际化的步伐。①

译文：① With the establishment of its Hong Kong manufacturing base as a milestone, ② Tong Ren Tang started from Beijing, expands in China and becomes international. ③ It now has business or services in 28 countries and regions in 5 continents, ④ helping internalize TCM. ②

分析：该段原文有两层意思，首先表明同仁堂走向全国和世界的标志性事件，然后说明目前的发展现状。为取得朗朗上口的修辞效果，文中运用平行结构"从'北京的同仁堂''中国的同仁堂'向'世界的同仁堂'跨越"，导致原文多次出现"同仁堂"。汉语简介中，有些重复是衔接的需要，有些是表达习惯问题，有些仅仅起到修辞作用，在翻译时需根据上下文适当调整。该简介译者根据句间逻辑关系，合并第①、②句话，直接译为"started from Beijing, expands in China and becomes international"，从而避免重复"同仁堂"一词，简洁但不失生动。

---

① 来源：https://www.tongrentang.com/article/70.html，搜索日期：2021－06－01。

② 来源：https://www.tongrentang.com/article/70.html，搜索日期：2021－06－01。

第四节　词语的翻译

汉英简介由于修辞习惯、意识形态和历史文化的不同,在词语使用方面有较大差异,在翻译过程中须基于差异对译文进行适当调整。

一、词语的对比分析

1. 修辞习惯

[**例1**]　① 学校在省属高校中拥有国家级重点学科<u>最多</u>,② 首批获得硕士、博士学位授权,首批设立博士后科研流动站,③ 首批成为国家"973"项目首席承担单位。①

原译:① Among all the colleges and universities in Shandong province, it <u>takes the lead</u> in the number of the state key disciplines, ② in offering master's and doctoral programs and post-doctoral research programs, ③ and also in undertaking the state "973 Projects" as a chief organization. ②

对比句:① Harvard faculty are engaged with teaching and research to push the boundaries of human knowledge. ② For students who are excited to investigate the biggest issues of the 21st century, Harvard offers an <u>unparalleled</u> student experience and a <u>generous</u> financial aid program, <u>with over $160 million</u> awarded to more than 60% of our undergraduate students. ③ The University has twelve degree-granting Schools in addition to the Radcliffe Institute for Advanced Study, offering <u>a truly global education</u>. ③

分析:中文简介有时在规模和档次上使用"最大""一流""最佳"等大词浓墨重彩地宣传自己(陈小慰,2017:175),如《山东中医药大学简介》原译第①句用"take the lead"表示学校一系列指标"处于全国同类院校前列"。西方的高校简介也使用大词,如哈佛医学院简介第②句中的"unparalleled""generous",第③句中的"global"等

---

① 来源:https://www.sdutcm.edu.cn/xxgk/xxjj.htm,搜索日期:2020-02-01。

② 来源:https://www.sdutcm.edu.cn/xxgk/English/Homepage.htm,搜索日期:2020-02-01。

③ 来源:https://hms.harvard.edu/about-hms,搜索日期:2020-07-30。

词语。但中英文简介使用大词的对象和方式有所不同。前者描述的对象是学校本身,缺少进一步解释说明;后者描述的对象是学校学生,并用"$160 million""60%"等数字和事实说明学生体验的丰富性、经济支持力度和教育国际化。

2. 意识形态

[**例2**]　①红色基因——诞生于广州这片中国近代与现代革命策源地的广药集团,始终与"红色血脉"紧紧相连,②培育了中国共产党早期领导人、广州起义的组织发动者、中央政治局常委杨殷,孙中山卫队长李朗如,中国"双百"人物向秀丽等革命先辈,③王老吉更曾为林则徐、毛泽东除病祛疾,留下佳话。红色血脉代代相传,④如今广药集团每年均开展纪念革命烈士、纪念向秀丽、纪念神农诞辰等传承红色基因主题活动,⑤并创新性地建立了"1+2+3+……"的大党建工作创新模式,即紧紧围绕以公司科学发展为中心,将党建工作与中医药公司特点相结合,继承与创新相结合,实现廉政建设创新、服务型党组织建设创新和党建运行方式创新等三个创新重点,促进党建工作与公司发展相互促进、不断创新,源源不断地为广药科学发展注入新鲜"活水"。①

原译:① GPHL, with its headquarters located in the cradle of Chinese revolutions in contemporary and modern times, has been a staunch supporter of CPC. ② It had produced a galaxy of revolutionaries, such as Yang Yin, a leader of CPC in early days, advocate and organizer of Guangzhou Uprising and member of the Standing Committee of the Political Bureau of the CPC Central Committee, Li Langru, Captain of Guards for Sun Yat-sen, and Xiang Xiuli, one of the 100 role models who have made great contributions to China since its founding with their touching deeds. ③ Besides, Wanglaoji Herbal Tea once cured Lin Zexu and Mao Zedong of their diseases, making it a household name. ④ To pass on the spirit of patriotism, GPHL organizes events in honor of revolutionary martyrs and Xiang Xiuli, and Shennong, the discoverer of medicine in the Chinese myth. ⑤ GPHL has built a new and innovative model of CPC development, focusing on the scientific development of the enterprise, taking into consideration the characteristics of traditional Chinese medicine enterprise, and integrating inheritance and innovation in corruption-free administration, service-oriented CPC organizations and CPC operation patterns, which has been promoting and innovating

---

① 来源:http://www.gpc.com.cn/aboutUs.html,搜索日期:2020 - 02 - 01。

the scientific development of both CPC and GPHL. [1]

　　分析：广药集团公司简介原译和中文简介内容完全一致,通过列举和广药集团相关的中国革命者的姓名和事迹,说明广药集团的革命传统,并增强公司的声誉。然而,对不了解中国革命史或对此不感兴趣的西方受众而言,这样的名人罗列没有太大意义。并且,逐句翻译会使受众感觉话语过于细碎,重点不清。

　　3. 口号式表达

　　[**例 3**]　① 立足于新时代新使命,同仁堂集团将以习近平新时代中国特色社会主义思想为指引,落实党的十九大和全国中医药大会精神,积极适应当前我国社会主要矛盾的新变化和广大群众对美好健康生活的新需求,② 推动工作重心由"服务疾病治疗为主"向"守护人民健康为主"的转变,③ 坚持稳中求进工作总基调,坚持"做精、做优、做强、做长"方针,坚持传承精华、守正创新,坚持以高质量党建引领高质量发展,积极实施"三步走"战略,④ 努力筑牢党建、质量、诚信三大基石,全力打造具有全球影响力的世界一流中医药大健康产业集团,努力实现"有健康需求的地方就有同仁堂"的战略愿景。[2]

　　原译：① Based on the new era and new mission, Beijing TRT Group will be guided by Xi Jinping's socialist ideology with Chinese characteristics in the new era and the spirit of the 19th National Congress of the Communist Party of China and the National Congress of traditional Chinese Medicine to keep abreast with the times and people's need in the new era. ② Its priority should transit from "medical services" to "promoting people's health". ③ It will stick to steady growth to improve, strengthen and refine its "three-phase" growth strategy for a high-quality development. ④ With Party building, quality and credibility as the three cornerstones, it aims to build a world-class TCM health group under the vision of serving people's health around the world. [3]

　　对比句：① With its vast reservoir of talent, extensive network of affiliates and commitment to problem solving, ② Harvard Medical School is uniquely positioned to steer education and research in directions that will benefit local, national and global communities. [4]

---

①　来源：http://en. gpc. com. cn/aboutUs. html,搜索日期：2020－02－01。

②　来源：https://www. tongrentang. com/article/70. html,搜索日期：2021－06－01。

③　来源：https://www. tongrentang. com/article/70. html,搜索日期：2021－06－01。

④　来源：https://hms. harvard. edu/about-hms,搜索日期：2020－07－30。

分析：中文简介中常用一些口号语，这与英语的行文习惯差别较大，翻译时我们需要首先对原文进行"瘦身"（张健、许天虎，2019：38）。同仁堂集团简介的结尾部分为目标愿景，原译受中文简介的影响，标语口号式的套语特征明显。对比句为哈佛医学院官网简介的结尾段，精练扼要、简短平实地表达了其目标愿景。

二、词语翻译的特点和策略

［**例4**］ ① 学校在省属高校中拥有国家级重点学科最多，② 首批获得硕士、博士学位授权，首批设立博士后科研流动站，③ 首批成为国家"973"项目首席承担单位。

改译：① Among all the colleges and universities in Shandong province, we take the lead in the number of the state key disciplines with 3 state key disciplines, 29 State TCM Administration key disciplines, etc., ② in offering master's and doctoral programs and post-doctoral research programs, ③ and also in undertaking the state "973 Projects" (a national key basic research development plan) as a chief organizer.

分析：在对原译进行翻译调整时，将第①句中的"takes the lead ... in the number ..."进行文字或数据上的补充（补充数据来源于原文），尽可能使话语平实有据。此外，第③句中"973"项目是国家重点基础研究发展计划，直译不能体现该项目的性质和重要地位，须进行补充解释。

［**例5**］ ① 红色基因——诞生于广州这片中国近代与现代革命策源地的广药集团，始终与"红色血脉"紧紧相连，② 培育了中国共产党早期领导人、广州起义的组织发动者、中央政治局常委杨殷，孙中山卫队长李朗如，中国"双百"人物向秀丽等革命先辈，③ 王老吉更曾为林则徐、毛泽东除病祛疾，留下佳话。红色血脉代代相传，④ 如今广药集团每年均开展纪念革命烈士、纪念向秀丽、纪念神农诞辰等传承红色基因主题活动，⑤ 并创新性地建立了"1+2+3+……"的大党建工作创新模式，即紧紧围绕以公司科学发展为中心，将党建工作与中医药公司特点相结合，继承与创新相结合，实现廉政建设创新、服务型党组织建设创新和党建运行方式创新等三个创新重点，促进党建工作与公司发展相互促进、不断创新，源源不断地为广药科学发展注入新鲜"活水"。

改译：① GPHL has been closely related to the Chinese history, with its headquarters located in Guangzhou, the cradle of Chinese revolutions in modern and contemporary times. ③ Wang Laoji, one of the staple products of GPHL, is even said to have helped cure Lin Zexu, a national hero, and Mao Zedong, the founder of the People's Republic of China. ④⑤ To pass on the spirit of patriotism, GPHL organizes events in honor of revolutionary martyrs, and further builds an innovative model of CPC development with its focus on constant innovation and sustainable development.

分析： 改译对内容进行了归纳整合,省译第②句,第③句只保留林则徐和毛泽东两个有代表性的例子。此外,党建部分属于国情,起不到信息、感染功能,因此对第④、⑤句进行整合,只保留实质性信息。

[**例 6**]　① 立足于新时代新使命,同仁堂集团将以习近平新时代中国特色社会主义思想为指引,落实党的十九大和全国中医药大会精神,积极适应当前我国社会主要矛盾的新变化和广大群众对美好健康生活的新需求,② 推动工作重心由"服务疾病治疗为主"向"守护人民健康为主"的转变,③ 坚持稳中求进工作总基调,坚持"做精、做优、做强、做长"方针,坚持传承精华、守正创新,坚持以高质量党建引领高质量发展,积极实施"三步走"战略,④ 努力筑牢党建、质量、诚信三大基石,全力打造具有全球影响力的世界一流中医药大健康产业集团,努力实现"有健康需求的地方就有同仁堂"的战略愿景。

改译： ① Guided by the Xi Jinping Thought on Socialism with Chinese Characteristics for a New Era, ② we transformed the mission of medical service into promoting people's health, ③ by inheriting the essence and maintaining the innovation. ④ We seek to create a world-class TCM health group and realize the vision of "Beijing TRT Group is where health begins".

分析： 改译时采取删除或释译的方法,淡化处理中文简介的意识形态色彩,让译文更贴近英语行文习惯。第①句省略了一些套语,保留了"习近平新时代中国特色社会主义思想"这一重要表述。第②~④句也进行了淡化处理,只保留了实质性信息。

第五节　翻译练习与任务

一、翻译练习

以下是中医药企事业单位网上简介部分内容,请根据英文简介规范进行必要的译前调整,并译成英语。

(1) 医院 2019 年门诊量 336 万人次,其中本部门诊量 236 万人次。本部开放住院床位 650 张。2011 年,医院受北京市大兴区政府委托,管理原大兴区中医医院,成立广安门医院南区。同时,医院积极推进区域医疗中心、医疗联合体建设,发挥中医药辐射北京市、京津冀和引领作用。

(2) 进入新时代,乘势谋发展。在习近平总书记对中医药提出的"传承精华,守正创新"重要指示精神的指导下,辽宁中医药大学坚定社会主义办学方向,坚持"立德树人"根本任务,秉持"厚德博学、继承创新"校训精神,全面推进内涵式发展,增强办学治校硬核实力,在推动辽宁全面振兴和祖国中医药事业传承发展中做出了重要贡献,正向着内涵丰富、特色优势突出的高水平中医药大学的奋斗目标扎实迈进,以新的更大成绩迎接中医药事业发展的美好明天!

(3) "同修仁德,济世养生"是同仁堂创立的初心,"全心全意为人民健康服务"是同仁堂不变的宗旨。同仁堂将"修合无人见,存心有天知""炮制虽繁必不敢省人工,品味虽贵必不敢减物力""但愿世间人无病,何惜架上药生尘"等古训内化为公司行为准则,造就了同仁堂"配方独特、选料上乘、工艺精湛、疗效显著"的制药特色,奠定了同仁堂质量和诚信文化的根基。

(4) 广安门原称广宁门,取广为安宁之意。甲子峥嵘岁月,广安门医院秉承"广安门护佑人民生活安宁康泰"的历史寓意,践行"广安广博、至精至诚"的院训精神,把"大医精诚"的核心价值观体现在医德医风上,转化为服务群众的理念,以病人为中心,以中医药特色为优势,努力为患者提供个性化、温馨化的优质中医药服务。把广安门医院建设成为优势突出、服务领先、管理科学、患者满意、员工幸福的中医国家队。

二、翻译任务

1. 下面是汉英对照《三亚市中医院简介》,请根据医药行业网上英文简介规范找出原译不妥之处,进行必要的内容和结构上的调整,讨论翻译过程中在语篇、段落、句子及词语层面所做的翻译调整、采取的翻译策略及原因。

医院简介

三亚市中医院始建于 1991 年,2008 年整体搬迁至凤凰路,占地 45 亩,总建筑面积 55 947.74 平方米。医院位于世姐选美赛址"美丽之冠"对面,面朝临春河,背靠虎豹岭,环境优雅,是一所集医疗、教学、科研、保健、康复、传统医药国际交流与合作为一体的三级甲等中医医院。截至 2014 年 12 月 31 日,全院总人数 592 人,其中博士 9 人,硕士 71 人,正高 14 人,副高 23 人。其中,全国名老中医专家、国务院特殊津贴专家 1 人,国家优秀中医临床研修人才 2 人,广州中医药大学博士研究生导师 1 人、硕士研究生导师 7 人。

医院拥有人员编制 635 人,编制床位 660 张。设职能科室 19 个,临床科室及医技科室 35 个,包括急诊、ICU、内、外、妇、儿、老年、骨伤、皮肤、男科、肛肠、针灸、推拿、康复、治未病、耳鼻喉科、口腔科、眼科、感染性疾病科、麻醉科、医学美容、影像、功能、检验、输血、中西药房等。其中国家临床重点专科 1 个(脾胃病科),国家中医重点专科 2 个(骨伤科、治未病中心),国家中医药管理局重点专科协作组单位 3 个(针灸科、临床药学、护理学),海南省重点专科 1 个(脑病专科)。

医院特色——"中医康复疗养游"

2002 年以来,医院突出中医特色,结合三亚得天独厚的自然环境和旅游资源,开设三亚欣欣荣中医疗养国际旅行社,率先在全国开展中医康复疗养游,截至 2014 年 12 月,已接待俄罗斯、瑞典、挪威、奥地利、德国、法国等国客人 40 余批,接待国外疗养包机 10 架次,为包括哈萨克斯坦总统纳扎尔巴耶夫、塔吉克斯坦总统拉赫默诺夫、俄罗斯联邦政府总理梅德韦杰夫等政要在内的 35 000 余位外宾提供高端定制健康服务。圆满完成俄罗斯别斯兰恐怖事件两批受伤儿童和 50 名吉尔吉斯斯坦儿童的中医康复疗养任务,获得由俄罗斯联邦政府总理签发的"为中俄友谊作出贡献"奖状、俄罗斯联邦卫生和社会发展部颁发的荣誉状,收到中华人民共和国外交部和吉尔吉斯斯坦驻华大使馆、塔吉克斯坦驻华大使馆的感谢信。

医疗康复、养生保健、健康服务、休闲度假于一体的新型健康产业项目,注重人们身体、心理和精神三个层面整体健康程度的提升,致力于打造中医药服务贸易国际化品牌,推动中医药健康服务贸易纵深发展。

医疗设备

医院配备 1.5 T 核磁共振、美国 GE 公司 innova3100 数字化平板血管机、16 层螺旋 CT、DR、SC2000 高端心脏彩色多普勒、多功能全身彩超、腹腔镜、关节镜、C 臂 X 光机、日立 7600 全自动生化分析仪、西门子移动式 DR 等进口系列先进设备,总价值 1.2 亿元。

医院文化

发展战略:中医有特色,西医上水平;中西医融会贯通,走现代中医之路。

核心价值:仁、和、精、诚。

院训：仁心精术，指仁爱之心，精湛之术。

院歌：《临春河畔的爱》。

服务宗旨："发扬中医、救死扶伤"。

医院荣誉

2007 年被评为"全国卫生系统先进集体"。

2008 年被批准为国家中医药管理局国际交流合作基地、对俄中医药合作协作组成员，被列为国家中医药服务贸易试点单位。

2009 年被评为"全国医药卫生系统先进集体""海南省中医医院先进单位"。

2011 年被评为"全国中医药文化建设先进单位"。

2012 年被评为"海南省文明单位"并通过国家中医药管理局三级甲等中医医院的评审。

2014 年被纳入国家首批中医药服务贸易先行先试骨干公司（机构）。

2014 年被评为全国"首届中医药科技推广工作先进集体"。

2014 年被海南省委、省人民政府授予海南省文明单位。

2014 年荣获"中国医疗机构公信力百家示范三甲医院"荣誉称号。

Sanya Traditional Chinese Medicine Hospital

Sanya Traditional Chinese Medicine Hospital is located on the opposite side of the building from the Beauty Crown Culture Centre (where the Miss World contest is held). The hospital faces the Linchun River and is near Fenghuang Mountain. It is a grade-A tertiary hospital offering medical care, education, research, healthcare services and International Chinese Medicine exchange and cooperation. As a new rural cooperative medical insurance and fixed-point unit of Hainan, the affiliated hospital of Guangzhou University of Chinese Medicine, the collaboration hospital of the First Affiliated Hospital of Guangzhou University of Chinese Medicine; the collaboration hospital of Guangdong Chinese Medicine Hospital, and the teaching hospital of Southern Medical University and Hainan Medical College. The hospital is the tele-medicine teaching center for the Liberation Army General Hospital (301 Hospital). It was authorized as the base of international exchange and cooperation by State Administration of Traditional Chinese Medicine of the People's Republic of China, it is also a national unit group member collaborating with Russia in traditional Chinese medicine, and a national experimental unit of Traditional Chinese Medicine Trade in Service, it was honored as the advanced collective of National Medicine Health System many times.

Sanya Traditional Chinese Medicine Hospital was founded in 1991, with the overall move to Fenghuang Rd. in 2008, the hospital covers about 30,000 m^2, the total construction area is 55,947.74 m^2. There is more than 600 staff, more than 40 people with senior professional titles, more than 70 people with intermediate professional titles, 8 doctors (including 2 postdoctoral) and 90 master postgraduate students. We have one person who regarded as an expert of the field of traditional Chinese medicine, and rewarded by the special allowance of the State Council. 2 national outstanding Chinese medicine clinical research and training talents, 6 Master candidate Supervisors in Guangzhou University of Chinese Medicine, and a base for postgraduate students.

There are more than 600 staff and 500 beds (there will be 660 beds and more than 750 staff when the third phase of our International Healthcare Centre project is completed, which will add 160 beds). The hospital consists of 13 administrative departments, 18 clinical departments, 8 medical and technology departments. The Orthopedic Department and the Spleen and Stomach Disease Department are China key-special units, the Cerebral Disease Department is a Hainan province key-special unit, and 2 Sanya key laboratories (Medical Biomechanics laboratory and spleen-stomach disease research laboratory), and an immune cells preparation section.

The hospital is well equipped with state-of-the-art medical apparatuses, such as a 1.5T MRI Scanner, a G.E. Innova 3100 DSA, 16-Slice CT, DR(Digital Radiography), SC2000 high-level cardiac color doppler, Digital Gastrointestinal Apparatus and Molybdenum Target X-ray, Multi-functions the whole body Ultrasonography, Laparoscope, Tris-dimension Traction Equipment, Mini-C-arm Fluotoscopy, TCD (Transcranial Doppler), Automatic Biochemical Analyzer, Laser Therapy Apparatus, Automatic Chinese Medicine Boiling-machine, etc. The total value is 120 million RMB.

Since 2002, Sanya Chinese Medicine Hospital has specialized in Traditional Chinese Medicine. It is the first hospital to carry out recuperation tourism of Traditional Chinese Medicine around the Country. Sanya Chinese Medicine Hospital has built Sanya Xin Xinrong TCM Healthcare Centre Intl. Travel Agency in the hospital, by using the unique environment and tourism resources available in Sanya. To date, we have provided treatment for more than 10 groups of foreign healthcare visitors from as far away as

Russia, Sweden, Norway, Austria, and other countries. We have chartered 10 foreign flights providing healthcare, and have offered treatment to more than 25 thousand visitors, and provided TCM therapy for two groups of injured Beslan children and 50 Kyrgyz children who suffered injuries in terrorist incidents. As a result, the Russian Federation government issued an award for "contributing to Sino-Russian friendship" to Sanya Chinese Medicine Hospital, and it received grateful letters from the Foreign Ministry of China and the Kyrgyz Republic embassy in China.

2. 广慈堂（Guang Ci Tang）是美国中成药领域的一个领导品牌。搜索广慈堂英文网上简介（https://www.activeherb.com/guang_ci_tang/），从语篇、段落和词语三个方面分析该简介及其传播效果。

三、扩展阅读

［1］刘季春.实用翻译教程（第三版）［M］.广州：中山大学出版社,2016.

［2］张健,许天虎.企业简介英译若干问题探讨［J］.上海翻译,2019（6）：36－40+28.

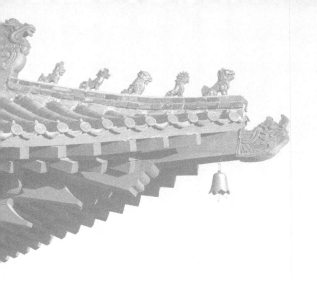

第八章
中医药公示语英译

公示语,也称标识语,是指公开面对公众,具有告示、指示、提示、显示、警示、标示功能,与生活、生产、生命、生态相关的文字及图形信息(戴宗显、吕和发,2005:38),类型包括标识、指示牌、路牌、标语、公告、提示语等(丁衡祁,2006:12)。公示语的覆盖面广泛,其翻译质量的优劣能够成为衡量国际化都市、国际旅游目的地语言环境和人文环境的重要依据,是一个地区、一个行业、一个国家形象的重要组成部分。国家医疗服务领域的汉语公示语及英译主要发挥服务信息功能,同时,作为具有呼吁、感召功能的一种文本(牛新生,2007:63),促使读者去行动、思考或感受,按照文本预期的功能做出反应。

第一节 语料导入

本章讨论所涉及的公示语包含图文语料和纯文字语料两种,图文语料用于第二节译例,包括商场、公园等公共场所及道路交通的常用公示语,还有部分疫情相关的公示语。第三节译例采取纯文字形式,主要来源于知网公示语相关论文。本节导入的语料限于图文语料,根据讨论时出现的先后顺序编号,英文语料在前,中文语料在后,纯文字语料将在第三节译例分析时一并呈现,不再单独列出。

一、英文语料

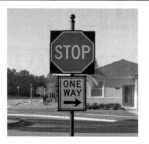 图 8-1	STOP ONE WAY 停！单行道！
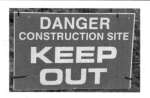 图 8-2	DANGER CONSTRUCTION SITE KEEP OUT 工地危险，请勿靠近！
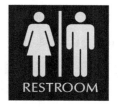 图 8-3	RESTROOM 卫生间
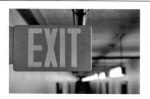 图 8-4	EXIT 出口
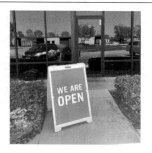 图 8-5	WE ARE OPEN 营业中

续　表

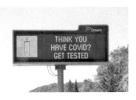 图 8 - 6	THINK YOU HAVE COVID? GET TESTED 觉得自己感染新冠了？核酸测一测！
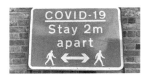 图 8 - 7	COVID-19 Stay 2m apart 防止新冠病毒传播，请保持 2 米间距！
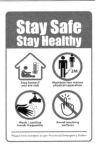 图 8 - 8	Stay Safe. Stay Healthy. Stay home if you are sick. Maintain two metres physical separation. Wash／sanitize hands frequently. Avoid touching surfaces. 防控勿忘，健康常伴！ 如有不适，请勿出门！保持 2 米社交距离！勤洗手！手勿触碰 表面！
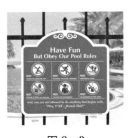 图 8 - 9	Have Fun. But Obey Our Pool Rules. NO! DIVING IN SHALLOW END NO! RUNNING, PUSHING, SHOVING NO! SWIMMING ALONE NO! PEEING IN POOL（Use Bathroom） NO! YELLING OR SCREEMING NO! GLASSWARE IN POOL AREA 好好享受，但请遵守泳池规则！ 禁止在浅水区跳水！禁止奔跑和推挤！禁止无人时游泳！禁止在 泳池内小便！禁止叫嚷和尖叫！禁止在泳池区域使用玻璃器皿！
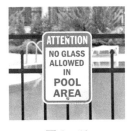 图 8 - 10	ATTENTION NO GLASS ALLOWED IN POOL AREA 注意！泳池区域禁止使用玻璃器皿！

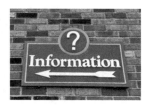

图 8－11

Information
咨询处

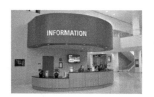

图 8－12

Information
咨询处

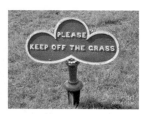

图 8－13

PLEASE KEEP OFF THE GRASS
请远离草地!

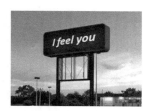

图 8－14

I feel you.
和你感同身受!

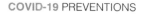
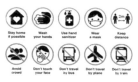

图 8－15

COVID-19 PREVENTIONS
Stay home if possible. / Wash your hands. /
Use hand sanitizer. / Wear a mask. / Keep distance. / Avoid crowd. /
Don't touch your face. / Don't travel by bus. / Don't travel by plane. / Don't travel by train.
新冠防护指南：非必要不出门/勤洗手/手部消毒/戴口罩/保持距离/不聚集/不触碰面部/不乘坐公共汽车/不乘坐飞机/不乘坐火车

续　表

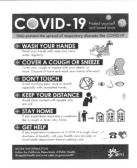

图 8-16

COVID-19
WASH YOUR HANDS／COVER A COUGH OR SNEEZE／DON'T TOUCH／KEEP YOUR DISTANCE／STAY HOME／GET HELP
新冠防护指南：勤洗手/咳嗽喷嚏捂口鼻/勿触碰面部/保持距离/非必要不出门/如有不适请及时寻求帮助（具体内容部分略）

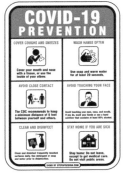

图 8-17

COVID-19 PREVENTION
COVER COUGHS AND SNEEZES ／ WASH HANDS OFTEN ／ AVOID CLOSE CONTACT／AVOID TOUCHING YOUR FACE／CLEAN AND DISINFECT／STAY AT HOME IF YOU ARE SICK
新冠防护指南：咳嗽喷嚏捂口鼻/勤洗手/保持适当距离/手勿触碰脸部/保持清洁勤消毒/生病期间不出门（具体内容部分略）

二、中文语料（包括原译）

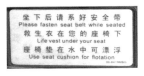

图 8-18

坐下后请系好安全带
救生衣在您的座椅下
座椅垫在水中可漂浮
Please fasten seat belt while seated.
Life vest under your seat.
Use seat cushion for flotation.
（摄于某航空公司,2023-03-02）

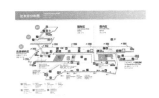

图 8-19

出发层分布图
Departures Level

191

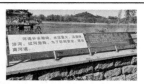 图 8-20	河道补水期间,水流量大、流速快,涉河、过河危险,为了您的安全,请远离河道。
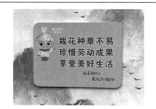 图 8-21	栽花种草不易 珍惜劳动成果 享受美好生活 (摄于上海陆家嘴滨江公园,2023-03-05)
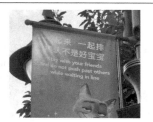 图 8-22	一起来,一起排,插队不是好宝宝 Stay with your friends and do not push past others while waiting in line. (摄于上海迪士尼,2023-06-01)
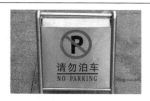 图 8-23	请勿泊车 NO PARKING
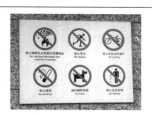 图 8-24	上海地铁站一公示牌(具体内容省略) (摄于上海地铁站,2023-02-19)
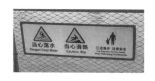 图 8-25	当心落水 当心滑跌 江边散步 注意安全 Danger! Deep Water Caution, Slip Pay Attention to Your Safety When Walk Along the Riverside. (摄于上海洋泾滨江,2023-02-19)

续 表

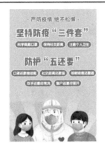 图 8-26	严防疫情 绝不松懈 坚持防疫"三件套" 防护"五还要"（具体略）
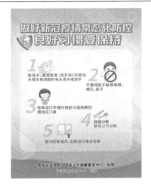 图 8-27	做好新冠疫情常态化防控,良好习惯要保持（具体略）

第二节　英语公示语文体特点

公示语表达简洁凝练,规范准确,以实现向公众提供告示、指示、提示、警告、限制、禁止、宣教等功能。汉英公示语的功能虽一致,但因汉语和英语在语言、文化、思维等方面的差异,公示语翻译实践存在诸多难点。为了译出更易于外籍人士理解的公示语,我们有必要先了解英语公示语的文体特点。本节将从词汇、句法、版面布置和图文匹配三个层面讨论英语公示语的文本特点,并进行汉英对比。

一、词汇层面

1. 英语公示语词汇特点

1）大写字母

大写字母具有正式、严肃的文体特点,能够快速提高目标受众对公示语内容的关注度。一般而言,引发的关注程度按照字母全部大写、字母大小写结合、所有首字母大写、仅句首字母大写的顺序逐渐减弱。

[例1] 警告、禁止类的"STOP""DANGER"(见图8-1、图8-2)

分析:这些公示语采用全大写的方式,传达非常明确的警告和禁止的意味。驾驶者遇到"STOP"停止标志却没停车,违反了交通安全的相关法规,要被处罚。如果因此产生更严重的后果,驾驶者承担全部责任。工地附近,或是任何一处有安全隐患的场所附近竖立的"DANGER"危险警告牌都具有强烈劝退的意味,如有任何人靠近,由此产生的危险或危害都需要自行承担结果。由此可见,通常容错率较小的情况,特别是涉及生命和法律法规的公示语会使用全部字母大写。

[例2] 明确指示类的"RESTROOM"和"EXIT"(见图8-3、图8-4)

分析:这类公示语没有禁止、警告的意味,但有时也会采用首字母大写。这类室内外指示性公示语采用大写的方式提高人们的关注度,使指示性更加明确,不会让人找错方向。其中"EXIT"也含有安全的意义,因为一般该出口在遇险或紧急情况下才使用。

[例3] 表达公示语发布者强烈的主观愿望或请求的"WE ARE OPEN"和"THINK YOU HAVE COVID? GET TESTED"(见图8-5、图8-6)

分析:这类公示语的发布者一般不是法律法规的制定者和执行者,可以是机构,也可以是企业。这些公示语非强烈警告,也非明确指示,只是告知和建议,从语气程度上来说仅使用首字母大写即可,但是"WE ARE OPEN"的发布者希望通过所有字母大写提高人们的关注度,传达在新冠疫情的特殊时期,在许多诊所都人满为患或关门歇业的情况下,坚持开门为周边居民服务的决心。同理,在高高的路牌上,"THINK YOU HAVE COVID? GET TESTED"除了在视觉上更能引起普通民众的关注之外,还传递了希望民众积极参加核酸检测的建议,凸显希望大家配合、团结抗疫的愿望。

[例4] 标题和内容在有限篇幅里结合(见图8-7、图8-8)

分析:这类公示语包含较多信息,大写部分起到标题的作用,可以提高人们的关注度,而内容部分采用常规的句子传达具体的信息。如图8-7所示,"COVID-19"作为最重要的信息载体全部大写,无疑能更好地抓人眼球,但其自身传达的信息很模糊,真正的信息是下面的"Stay 2m apart",提醒人们保持2米以上的社交距离。图8-8在放大"Stay Safe""Stay Healthy"字体的同时,每个单词首字母大写,吸引注意力,同时语气委婉,增强了劝告和宣教指导的功能。由此可见,当公示语所包含的细节信息比较多的时候,标题和细节、重点和次要点通过大小写相结合,在有限的篇幅中相互协调,凸显重点。

[例 5]　对公示语效果的期待(见图 8 - 9、图 8 - 10)

分析：图 8 - 9 中，"Have Fun But Obey Our Pool Rules"体现出管理者在标题上不希望语气太强硬，引起游客的不满，因此除了语言用"Have Fun"之外，每个单词只有首字母大写，使得提醒的意味多于强制，容易使人接受；反观下面的内容全部大写，因其会危及生命，因此显示出强烈的禁止意味。有趣的是，在"NO! PEEING IN POOL (Use Bathroom)"公示语中，全部字母大写表达了严禁的意思，而括号里的"使用卫生间"采用了首字母大写，表示这是建议而非强制。图 8 - 10 采用了全部大写的方式，标题即信息，管理者借此郑重地告诫游客遵守管理规定，希望游客人人自觉。

总之，公示语发挥其功能的基础和前提是吸引受众的注意力，因此公示语大写的情况日趋普遍，尤其是禁止、警告、限制、迫使等语气强烈的公示语。一般而言，选择全部字母大写还是首字母大写，或是两者结合，取决于多种因素，包括公示语字数和展示面积、公示语的功能和管理者的主观愿望等，这些因素也会相互影响并最终决定公示语的呈现。

2）名词和名词词组

英语公示语，尤其是具有指示和告知功能的公示语，又称静态公示语，大量使用名词和名词词组。简短凝练的名词和名词词组让人很容易抓住公示语传达的关键信息(谢丹，2017：34)，如"Toll Station""Registration Office""Emergency Room"。此外，像"Waiting Room""Parking"这样的公示语，虽然其动名词形态使之带有动词性质，但是这类动名词的名词属性要强于动词属性，故可以归入名词范围。

[例 6]　指向型和指示型的差异(见图 8 - 11、图 8 - 12)

分析：同样是表示"咨询处"的公示语，图 8 - 11 的公示语是指向型的，指向"咨询处"这个地点的行进方向，而图 8 - 12 的公示语是指示型的，指出了这个地方就是"咨询处"所在。有时候，为了方便区别，指向型的公示语配合箭头指明方向，而指示型的公示语会加上表示属性的名词，如"information desk"等。同样，医院里有很多公示牌也存在此类差异。如表示 CT 检查室的标牌，有时是"CT"，有时是"CT RM"，前者表示指向功能，而后者指明这个空间的使用属性。所以在翻译过程中，译者应该首先明确该公示语的类型和功能。

3）动词原形和动名词

静态公示语大量使用名词(组)，而使用动词和动名词的公示语又称动态公示语(谢丹，2017：35)，更适合用于劝告、迫使、强制和禁止的功能，而且公示语常见的祈使句的语法要求使动词成为公示语的又一鲜明特点。

[**例7**] 动词原型的使用(见图8-2、图8-6~图8-8)

分析：英语公示语动词原型的使用常见于表达请求、迫使、警告等功能。如图8-2中的"KEEP OUT"警告开车经过的人避让工地；图8-6中的"GET TESTED"建议和请求人们主动进行核酸检测；图8-7中的"Stay 2m apart"迫使人们保持适当的距离；图8-8"Stay Safe. Stay Healthy."警告人们不聚集，同时建议了具体的防疫措施。

[**例8**] 动名词的使用(见图8-9)

分析：动名词常常和"No"连用，表达禁止、警告和请求(梅美莲、杨仙菊，2013：59)。如图8-9中，"NO! DIVING IN SHALLOW END""NO! RUNNING, PUSHING, SHOVING""NO! SWIMMING ALONE""NO! PEEING IN POOL(Use Bathroom)""NO! YELLING OR SCREAMING""NO! GLASSWARE IN POOL AREA"，表达严禁的强烈语气。此外惊叹号和大写字母更增加了"严禁"的意味。因其强烈的严肃性，这类公示语常使用在涉及生命安全，涉嫌违法警告的公示语中。

2. 汉英公示语词汇特点对比

[**例9**] 大小写上的差异(见图8-18)

分析：汉语没有大小写之分，但国内中文公示语下面基本都有英译，在翻译汉语公示语时，译者可以酌情考虑译文的大小写问题，亦可对管理者提出自己的意见和建议。图8-18空间比较局促，因此采用第一个单词首字母大写(这种方法对于句子形式的公示语尤为适用)，也可以每个单词首字母大写。

[**例10**] 名词指示型公示语中指向和属性上的差异(见图8-19)

分析：指示型公示语是公示语的重要组成部分，日常生活中最为多见。指示功能的汉语公示语同时包含了指向的功能和该空间的物理属性，而英语公示语视情况而定，更注重公示语的功能属性和信息内涵。如图8-19中，"出发层分布图"带有表示属性的"图"，虽然该字没有指示功能意义，但习惯使然。而在英语相对应的公示语中，通常不带"图"。因此，该词在英译中可以省译。此外，像"游客通道""旅客通道"之类的公示语，直接译为"Visitors"和"Passengers"即可。当然，有些如"Restrooms"之类的合成词，汉英并无差别，已经包括了指向和属性。

[**例11**] 在表达"严禁"或"禁止"等功能时的表达差异(见图8-20)

分析：汉语公示语在表达警告和劝告时，受礼仪之邦的传统影响，期望以理服人，让受众对后果了然，自觉遵守公示语传达的信息。如图8-20首先说明设牌的原因是"河道补水期间，水流量大，流速快"，指明"涉河、过河危险"大，警告可能发生的危害生命的后果，随后说明发布公示语的目的，提出警告或劝告。但是，英语公示语通常直指所要求的行为本身,类似"DANGER: KEEP AWAY FROM RIVER"。因此,在汉英翻译中,直接表明公示语禁止、劝诫或迫使的行为信息是比较符合英语公示语的表达习惯的。

[**例 12**]　诗歌体公示语的英译(见图 8－21)

分析:诗歌体经常出现在表达"劝告"的汉语公示语中,典型的就是公园绿化公示语,比如图 8－21 中的"栽花种草不易,珍惜劳动成果,享受美好生活"。但英语公示语并没有类似的谆谆劝导,可将之译为"Please Keep Off the Grass",表达直白,但信息明确。甚至有些警告型的公式语也会采用诗歌体的形式,比如交通安全类的"道路千万条,安全第一条""河水无情,生命无价"等等,朗朗上口,便于记忆。这类汉语特色的公示语英译应遵循英语公示语的表达习惯,精简内容。

二、句子层面

1. 英语公示语句法特点

1)常见句型

[**例 13**]　祈使句(见图 8－2、图 8－6~图 8－9、图 8－13)

分析:祈使句是英语公示语常用的句型。该句型所表达的请求、劝告、迫使、警告、禁止等功能用以促使或限制某一行为的发生,和公示语的功能契合度非常高,因此祈使句在公示语中的占比非常高,比如图 8－2 的"KEEP OUT",图 8－6 的"GET TESTED",图 8－7 的"Stay 2m apart",图 8－8 的"Stay Safe. Stay Healthy.",图 8－9 的"Obey Our Pool Rules"和图 8－13 的"PLEASE KEEP OFF THE GRASS"。

[**例 14**]　陈述句(见图 8－5、图 8－14)

分析:除了祈使句,陈述句也是公示语常用句型之一,用于表达告知和提醒。和祈使句相比,陈述句的公示语语气显得稍弱,但更正式,更类似于法律法规条款。陈述句更合适"感染型"功能的公示语,如图 8－5"WE ARE OPEN"和图 8－14"I feel you",加上第一人称和第二人称的使用,使公示语发挥更好的渲染作用。

2)时态[例 1]

[**例 15**]　一般现在时(见图 8－5、图 8－14)

分析:一般现在时是英语公示语的常见时态(谢丹,2017:37),因为公示语表达的内容一般具有普世价值,或在某一种文化内具有稳定的特性,因此一般现在时最能显示公示语的不以个人意志为转移的客观属性。不仅如此,公示语的功能也决定了公示语对受众传达的信息是"当下的""即时的",也是"普遍的""持久有效"的概念,所以一般现在时也是最佳的时态选择,如图 8-5 和图 8-14 所示。

3）语态

[**例 16**]　主动态和被动态的使用（见图 8-5、图 8-10）

分析：主动态和被动态在英语公示语中都比较常见,根据公示语的不同功能而定。由于被动态能隐去施动者,突出行为事件,显得更为正式和严肃,适合"告知"和"提醒"的功能,让受众更关注所传达的信息,而不是传达信息的主体。如图 8-10 "NO GLASS ALLOWED IN POOL AREA"采用了被动态,公示语发布者希望游客关注点放在"泳池区域严禁使用玻璃器皿"这个行为,而不是公示语发布者,因为玻璃器皿一旦破碎,会对游客的人身安全造成极大的威胁。相比较而言,主动态能更好地引起共情,增加感染性,而且指向性更明确,如图 8-5 所示,虽然"OPEN"就可以表达"营业中"的意思,但"WE ARE OPEN"更能体现出和大家一起渡过难关的人文关怀。

2. 汉英公示语句法特点对比

[**例 17**]　英语的形合和汉语的意合（见图 8-13、图 8-21、图 8-22）

分析：汉英公示语都倾向于使用短句,契合了公示语要求语言简明易懂（张小萌、李芳,2022）,能快速有效地吸引注意力,并完成所要传达的信息这一特点。但汉英公示语在句型结构上存在明显差异:汉语句子结构是"意合型",通过意义衔接;而英语属于"形合",通过我们熟知的语法手段保持连贯（谭益兰,2013：62）。如图 8-21 中的三句公示语,"栽花种草不易"讲述绿化工作的艰辛,所以要"珍惜劳动成果",大家才能"享受美好生活",从汉语的"意合"角度看是非常流畅的。但假如我们用英语的"形合"将这句话直译出来,译文会冗长、生硬,不符合英语公示语的特点。所以一般此类汉语公示语都可以借鉴英语的"Please keep off the grass"进行翻译,如图 8-13 所示。再如图 8-22 中公示语"一起来,一起排,插队不是好宝宝",这个例子再次让我们看到汉英两种语言在结构上的差异给翻译带来的困难。原译文"Stay with your friends and do not push past others while waiting in line"分为了两个小句子,用一个肯定句和一个否定句明确地指出"该做"和"不该做"的行为,虽少了原句的俏皮,但公示语英译的第一原则是功能性,即将公示语的信息用受众能理解并接受的方式传达出去,而不是一味追求"原汁原味"。

三、版面布置和图文匹配

1. 英语公示语版式特点

符号学的发展促使标志和符号在全球范围内传播和统一,是公示语实现无障碍沟通的重要基础。此外,全球化使人们的交流日益增多,出国旅行和工作也日益普遍,促使具有普遍意义的图片和符号在公示语中大量使用。图片和符号在公示语中可以不依赖文字,或和文字相结合,更好地发挥公示语的各种功能。图片和符号优于文字的特点是生动、形象、具体、易懂。当然很多抽象概念还无法用简单的图片呈现,所以文字还是公示语的重要组成部分,但是图文结合会越来越多地应用于公示语。

[**例 18**] 图片和符号的结合(见图 8-15、图 8-16)。

分析:图文结合在英语公示语中非常普遍。如图 8-15,易懂的图标、短小的句子,清晰地传达出人们应该采取何种措施保护自己。从尺寸大小看,图标要明显大于文字。图 8-16 中,大写的字母和放大的字体已经能明确传达防疫的信息,但是在其右边仍配有一些简笔画来吸引人们的注意。图片能使公示语的普及性得到延伸,使不同识读水平、文化背景的人都能接收到公示语所传达的信息(张小萌、李芳,2022:1048)。

[**例 19**] "禁停"标志中图片和符号的使用(见图 8-23~图 8-25)

分析:现在街头常见的禁停公示牌如图 8-23 所示,信息明确,下面还配有汉语和英语。而且,画面中"P"占据了中心位置,凸显以符号和图片为主、文字为辅的特点。这样的公示语在街头小巷越来越普遍,特别是公共交通公示语(如图 8-24)、公共设施附近的公示语和旅游景点附近的标识语(如图 8-25)。

2. 汉英公示语版式特点对比

[**例 20**] 汉英公示语图文使用的异同(见图 8-15、图 8-16、图 8-17、图 8-26、图 8-27)

分析:如前例所示,汉语公示语的图形元素在不断增多,尤其是交通标志,几乎和英语公示语差异不大。但在其他公示语方面,汉英公示语的图片使用存在一些差异。首先,汉语没有大写,所以汉语的标题和内容通过放大字号或改变字形和颜色加以区分(见图 8-26、图 8-27)。其次,在图片和文字的关联性方面,英语公示语(如图 8-15、图 8-16、图 8-17)的图片和文字在数量上倾向于一一对应的关系,在内容上图片和文字的匹配度较高,且在版面上图片的占比不小,有的还超过了文字的面积(如图 8-15、图 8-17)。这样的设置和安排有利于公示语信息更高效、更广泛地传播。汉语公示语倾向于使用文字,配图更多是对整个公示语的信息表达,但是汉语公示语也在悄然发生改变(如图 8-27)以更利于信息的传播。因此,为了最大可能地发挥公示语的功能,译者除了在语言翻译上下功夫,在呈现方式上也须更符合英语使用者的习惯。

第三节　翻译原则和策略

本节聚焦中医院和新冠疫情防控公示语,基于公示语英译的凝练性、协调性和交际性原则,分析公示语英译存在的问题,并进行相应的翻译调整。

一、语言凝练

公示语使用的场景是公共场所,决定了人的注意力在公示语上停留的时间是有限的,所以公式语要言简意赅,最快最直接地传达涉及的信息。由于汉、英属于两种完全不同的语言形式,两种语言在思维方式和语言表达上存在很大差异。汉语多用意合法,句子短小精悍,而英语多用形合法,句子比较长。汉语公示语的诗歌体特征在感染型的公示语上体现得更为典型。因此英译这类公示语时,英文的句子会大大长于汉语公示语,不够凝练,很难让受众瞬间领会公示语的要义,削弱了公示语的交际功能。当遇到汉语公示语语义重复、表达繁复时,译者可以适当进行精简。

[**例1**]　小儿推拿外治诊室

原译: Small Kids' External Treatment with Massage Room①

改译: Pediatric Tuina (Physiotherapy) Room

分析: 推拿是中医外治手法之一,所以汉语中的"推拿外治"只需译出"推拿"即可。《公共服务领域英文译写规范》将"推拿"和"按摩"分别译为"tuina"和"massage"。推拿和按摩是两个不同的概念。虽然外籍患者可能对按摩"massage"更为熟悉,但是假如把"推拿"和"按摩"混为一谈,显然不利于推拿这一中医特色外治方法的对外传播。且"tuina"的译法已经越来越普遍,为人所知晓和接受。如果担心外籍患者看不懂,可以增译"physiotherapy"作为解释性说明(王畅、杨玉晨,2018:42)。"Small Kids"口语化的表达不符合公示语规范性要求,也不够凝练,使用"pediatric"一词更符合英语的使用习惯。

[**例2**]　患者至上,救死扶伤

原译: PUT THE PATEINTS ABOVE EVERYTHING. HEAL THE WOUNDED

---

①　选自:王畅,杨玉晨.生态翻译学视角下 TCM 医院公示语英译研究[J].上海翻译,2018(4):39-43.

AND RESCUE THE DYING^①

改译：Your health is our priority.

分析：原译文完整地指出了汉语公示语的意义，语言表达和结构符合英语习惯，可以向外籍患者传递医院的医学精神和人文关怀，但是译文过长，且全部采用大写字母，一定程度上减慢了阅读速度，比起中文公示语，翻译显得冗长，不够简练。此外，英语公示语，特别是感染型的公示语，常用到第一人称和第二人称，以拉近和患者之间的距离，让患者产生更强的代入感，而中文公示语通常使用无人称泛指任何第三人，距离感比较大。因此，建议改译为"Your health is our priority"，其语言长度和原文相近，同时也可以体现汉语公示语传达的以人为本、病人为先的人文精神。

[**例3**] 应检尽检、应收尽收、应治尽治

原译：make sure all patients are examined, admitted to hospitals and treated^②

改译：Assure people are tested and patients treated

分析：汉语公示语喜欢使用四字词语和排比，英语公示语常见的修辞是押韵、双关语等。所以假如在形式上翻译成英语排比，会增加难度和中式英语的嫌疑。"make sure all patients are examined, admitted to hospitals and treated"的译文重点放在"检""收""治"三个动词上，把句子的排比改为句子内部词组的排比，符合英语的表达方式，语言表达较为简洁。但是仔细分析发现，该英译还有更简练的空间。首先，把三个动词的主语归为"all patients"值得商榷，因为"检"的对象是所有需要参加检测的人员，确诊后才能归为"病人"。其次，就该翻译本身而言，"admit to hospitals"为词组，改为"hospitalize"可以更简洁。考虑到"hospitalized"和"treated"本身有意义上的重合，建议翻译一方即可。

[**例4**] "预防千万条，口罩第一条""口罩你不戴，病毒把你爱""口罩戴得快，病毒说拜拜"^③

译文：wear a covering mask

分析：这些汉语公示语表达诙谐，读来朗朗上口，容易口口相传，让人印象深刻，但是英语语言使用者很难理解和欣赏其中的诙谐和对仗。在英译的过程中，表达出汉语公示语的核心内容——戴好口罩即可。

---

① 选自：丁杨，孔祥国.北京市中医医院标识语英译的现状与对策[J].中医药导报，2015，21（5）：103－106.

② 选自：陈柯，张瑜.论防控新型冠状肺炎中英公示语的翻译等值问题[J].宁波工程学院学报，2020，32（2）：53－56.

③ 选自：王新.新冠肺炎疫情下的标语研究[J].山西大同大学学报（社会科学版），2020，34（2）：109－114.

二、文化协调

协调指的是文化层面翻译的归化现象,竭力创造自然流畅的译文,既展现中医药文化的内涵,又创造符合目标语言文化习惯的表达。由于中西方文化传统、行为规范等不同,如处理不当,译文容易引起误解。中医在哲学基础、治疗理念、药材选用等诸多方面与西医存在巨大差异,因此中医医院标识语英译更需要关注文化因素,积极对外传播中医药文化。

[**例5**] 治未病中心

原译: preventive treatment center①

改译: TCM Preventive Treatment Center / TCM Health Management Center

分析:"治未病"的概念是中医健康文化的核心内容之一,对于传播中医文化有着重要的意义。"治未病"指采取相应措施维护健康,防止疾病的发生与发展。"未病"是一种亚健康状态,不是某种具体疾病的意思,可见"治未病"的重点在于"防",所以翻译为"preventive treatment center"体现了"预防于未然"的意义,但是还应考虑到"preventive treatment"和西医的"preventive medicine"(预防医学)比较接近,可能会使外籍患者产生错误的理解,认为两者是相同的。但实际上西医所讲的预防医学和中医治未病是两个不同的概念。预防医学的主要研究对象是传染病和流行病,和中医治未病是完全不同的概念。改译通过增译 TCM,用以明确中医特色概念。

[**例6**] 名老中医工作室

原译: Distinguished Veteran TCM Specialist Studio / Retired TCM Master Clinic②

改译: Senior TCM Specialist Clinic

分析:把工作室翻译为"studio"不恰当。因为虽然"studio"有"室"的含义,在语义上实现了汉英对等,但是"studio"一般指艺术家工作场所的工作室,不符合原文中医生工作室的意义,改为"clinic"比较合适。"veteran"在英语中有"退伍老兵"的意义,和原文的医生职业不符合。而"retired"也有不妥之处,因为在英语文化中年龄是一个比较敏感的词,"retired"恰恰暴露出了这个问题。在中国文化中有"中医越老越吃香"的说法,表示患者对医生资历和经验的看重,但是在英语文化中更推崇"年富力强",建议用

---

① 选自:王畅,杨玉晨.生态翻译学视角下 TCM 医院公示语英译研究[J].上海翻译,2018(4):39-43.

② 选自:宋世豪,童林,朱文晓.浅析目的论视域下中医院公示语英译原则——以郑州3所中医院为例[J].中国校外教育,2018(11):95-96.

"senior"代替"retired",体现对长者医生的尊重,也体现出名老中医资历深厚、经验丰富的特点。再者,"distinguished"和"specialist"都含有资深的意义,略显重复,保留一个即可。

三、交际功能的实现

医院公示语英译的交际性指翻译文本的社会属性,译文应以让外籍患者接收到同样内容的信息为第一要求,让患者获得方便快捷的就医体验,并体验同种程度的感召力,从而采取预期的行为。

[例7]　疮疡门诊①

译文:Skin Ulcers Clinic

分析:医院公示语的对象是普通患者,公示语英译应该以满足普通外籍患者的就医需求为目标,重点突出公示语的交际功能。公示语英译要避免使用远高于普通外籍患者认知的冷僻词或专业性较强的术语。根据疾病的定义,疮疡是指各种致病因素侵袭人体后引起的一切体表化脓感染性疾病的总称,而英语疾病描述中,"skin ulcers"表述为"A skin ulcer is a crater-like, open sore on the skin. The wound is roughly circular, the center of which is open and raw. ... skin ulcers cause a crater-like depression in the skin, which may weep clear fluid (called serous), blood, or, when infected, pus. The outer border of a skin ulcer is often raised and inflamed"②. 这两者的表述虽不完全相同,但比较接近,根据《公共服务领域英文译写规范》规定,公示语翻译应"尽量使用英语国家同类信息的习惯用语",所以把"疮疡门诊"译为"Skin Ulcers Clinic"能更容易被外籍患者理解,更好地发挥源公示语的交际功能。如将"疮疡"翻译为"suppurative infection",虽然在语义上能做到信息对等,但是在实际使用过程中交际性不强。

[例8]　肛肠科

原译:Anal & Intestinal Department③

改译:TCM Proctology Department

分析:在公示语英译中,还应考虑译文是否符合公示语"文明性"的要求(孙小春,2020:41),避免因为使用不雅词汇,甚至禁忌语,使外籍患者产生心理不适感。

---

① 选自:丁杨,孔祥国.北京市中医医院标识语英译的现状与对策[J].中医药导报,2015,21(5):103-106.

② 来源:https://www.verywellhealth.com/skin-ulcers-overview-4175813,搜索日期:2023-04-05.

③ 选自:宋世豪,童林,朱文晓.浅析目的论视域下中医院公示语英译原则:以郑州3所中医院为例[J].中国校外教育,2018(11):95-96.

比如在"肛肠科"的翻译中,要尽量避免"anus""ass"等相关禁忌语,所以原译使用"anal"一词较为不妥(宋世豪、童林、朱文晓,2018:96)。此外,"intestinal"意为"小肠的",而非肛肠科的诊疗范围,是为错译。《中华人民共和国国家标准》和世界中医药学会联合会在翻译"肛肠"时都采用了"Proctology"一词。考虑到中医肛肠科除了常用的手术手法,还有外用药和坐浴等特色疗法,不妨增译 TCM 以体现中医特色。因此,建议将肛肠科译为"TCM Proctology Department"。

[例9] 勤消毒

译文:Clean and Disinfect

分析:"勤消毒"是疫情防控的有效措施之一。如果将"勤消毒"直译为"Keep sterilizing",可能会引发"不停消毒"的误会,从而导致因消毒不当而存在的危险。该防疫公示语主要的功能是指导人们如何保护自己,因此建议不妨改为"Clean and Disinfect",既避免"keep"导致理解和操作上的歧义,又能起到防护指导作用,而且在国外的宣传公示语也常用"Clean and Disinfect"这样的表述。

第四节　翻译练习与任务

一、翻译练习

按照汉语公示语英译规范,将下列公示语译为英文。

(1) 就诊区

(2) 住院区

(3)(急诊)分诊台

(4)(普通)分诊台/门诊接待室

(5) 划价处

(6) 取药处/药房

(7) 隔离门诊

(8) 发热筛查室

(9) 医患关系部

(10) 肺病门诊

(11) 中医科

（12）中医消化门诊

（13）中医皮肤门诊

（14）中医儿科

（15）中医妇科

（16）中医耳鼻喉科

（17）中医骨病治疗科

（18）中西医结合科

（19）传统敷贴室

（20）体质医学门诊

（21）中草药小包装调剂室

（22）国医堂

（23）现在的不见面是为了以后更长久的相聚

（24）早发现、早报告、早隔离、早治疗

（25）家庭保持通风，讲究卫生别乱跑

二、翻译任务

1. 以下图片包含了某城市颁布的《新"七不"规定》和英译。以小组为单位讨论和分析这些公示语英译是否恰当，存在哪些问题，如何修正，并阐述理由。

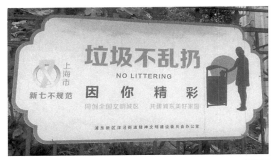
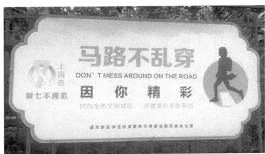
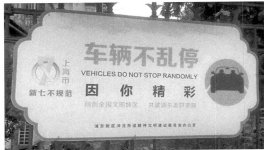
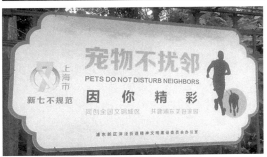

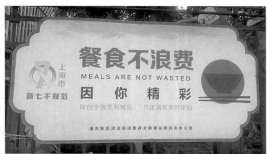
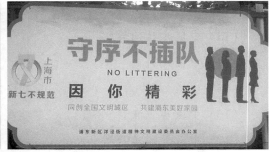
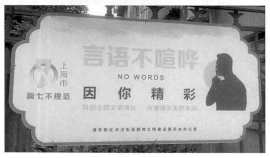

2. 中医博大精深,源远流长,产生了许多中医流派和特色专科,比如以"石氏伤科""徐氏儿科""朱氏妇科"等为代表的海派中医。请以小组为单位,讨论、分析这些招牌公示语的英译,并归纳和总结此类招牌公示语的翻译方法。

三、扩展阅读

[1] 谢丹. 变译在公示语汉英翻译中的应用[M]. 成都:西南交通大学出版社,2017.

[2] 王畅,杨玉晨. 生态翻译学视角下 TCM 医院公示语英译研究[J]. 上海翻译,2018(4):39－43.

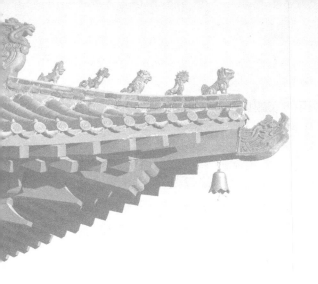

第九章
中医药外宣
翻译工作坊

全球化背景下的中医药外宣已经不仅仅是针对单个文本的翻译,更多的是基于多文本、多平台、多模态、即时性、结构化的翻译项目,很可能是某个中医馆印制的产品和治疗手册、宣传页、官方网站、类似微信公众号等新媒体同步发布的内容;还可能需要翻译成英语、日语、法语等多国语言;也可能是某一本厚厚的中医类科普书籍需要翻译,还附带教学视频、宣传资料或网站等。不难发现,现代的中医药外宣翻译对象可以是"除文学翻译之外的所有应用文体"(高芸,2023:10),包括但不限于典籍文献、政府文书、新闻文本、科普文本、科研论文、中医药产品说明资料或商务广告、中医药机构网站等。这类大型翻译项目字数多、格式复杂、交付时间要求高,必然需要多译员合作,综合应用各类翻译技术,并引入翻译项目经理的有效管理,才能高质高效完成。这类项目已经不是传统翻译的理念和技术所能处理的,而这正和目前翻译行业走向现代语言服务行业①的趋势不谋而合。

现代语言服务行业的商业化特质注定了翻译需求有别于之前的传统翻译,其中有个特别的概念——GILT。CILT 是"Globalization""Internationalization""Localization""Translation"这四个单词的首字母组合的缩写,即"全球化、国际化、本地化和翻译"。这四个过程是使产品进入全球市场而进行的技术和市场活动,包括全球化战略、国际化设计、本地化集成、语言翻译等紧密联系的系列过程。中医药文化或产品要走出去,就需要我们讲述中国故事,传播中医药文化,进行中医药商务活动,也需要针对特定国别语言和文化进行加工,使之适应多种语言、文化习俗以及特定区域市场,此谓

---

① 中国翻译协会将语言服务业定义为提供跨语言、跨文化信息转换服务和产品,以及相关技术研发、工具应用、知识管理、教育培训等专业化服务的现代服务业。

中医药的全球化、国际化和本地化，亦即中医药外宣翻译的核心目的：推动中医药文化在海外广泛传播，促进世界对中医药文化深入了解，树立正向、全面的中医药文化形象，从而助推中国良好国际形象的建立。

在这样的背景下，中医药外宣翻译人才的培养目标已不仅仅是培养单纯的文本翻译人才，更应该着力于培养高层次、应用型、专业性的中医药翻译人才，不仅仅要学习语言和翻译基础，还需要掌握各类翻译技术，熟悉理解实际的翻译项目操作流程，并且掌握该流程中各个角色所需要的技能，以更好地满足客户的翻译需求。"中医药外宣翻译工作坊"课程正是契合现代语言服务行业的人才培养要求，依托真实的翻译项目而进行的实践操作型课程。整个教学过程分为三个阶段——译前、译中以及译后。学生通过试译分为两组，即练习组和项目组。每组学生分为项目经理、译员、审校三类角色，在教师指导下，通过使用 CAT（Computer Aided Tools，计算机辅助翻译软件）工具的支持协作完成每个阶段的不同身份所对应的具体任务。每项任务关联了翻译能力构成中的一项或多项子能力。项目经理能够培养全面的翻译职业能力，译员和审校能在双语语言能力、翻译认知和翻译策略选择能力方面获得充分的训练，然后通过项目协作流程以及课堂分享汇报互相学习，既体现"专业化"，也体现"职业化"，在语言与翻译技能学习的基础上进行真实中医药外宣翻译项目的实践。

第一节　翻译项目概述

一、项目介绍

1）**原文名称**：《新冠肺炎中医防治读本》
2）**出版信息**：作者：严世芸
　　　　　　　出版社：上海科学普及出版社
　　　　　　　出版时间：2020 年 2 月
　　　　　　　ISBN：9787542777348
3）**原文语言**：简体中文
4）**原文格式**：PDF
5）**原文字数**：22 963 字

6）**目标语言**：美式英语

7）**工作方式**：基于单机版软件的翻译项目协作

8）**项目周期**：21 天

二、任务要求

1）**学员分组**：共分 2 组（练习组和项目组）,5 人/组

2）**角色分工**：项目经理、译员、审校

3）**翻译软件**：memoQ 软件

4）**项目经理**：

• 设计和撰写翻译协作方案（包括任务分析、角色分工、流程安排、时间安排等）

　• 创建项目

　• 分配任务

　• 监督进度

　• 回收任务

　• 合成译文

　• 导出译文

　• 撰写项目总结与反思、提交所有要求的项目文件

5）**译员和审校**：

　• 接收任务

　• 完成翻译或审校工作

　• 交付任务

　• 软件翻译或审校功能应用

　• 问题解决

6）**交付要求**：

　• 翻译协作方案（成员分工流程及时间节点表、风格指南、术语表）

　• 每个小组总的项目文件+协作过程文件+个人项目文件+个人总结

　• 排版后的译文文件（Word 和 PDF 各一份）

三、项目参与者

教师在上海中医药大学二年级中医药翻译硕士生（MTI,2020 级和 2021 级）中分

别实施了该翻译项目。在项目开始前,教师组织试译,要求学生在规定时间内翻译一段 800 字左右的相关内容,并由两位审校老师匿名打分,按照分数高低将学生分为练习组和项目组。项目组要提交给客户定稿译文,而练习组只参与整个项目翻译流程,无需承担最终成果交付的责任。2020 级和 2021 级中医药翻译硕士生项目组以下分别简称"2020 级项目组"和"2021 级项目组"。

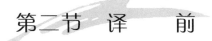

第二节 译 前

译前可以分为项目计划、项目执行中的预处理和译前准备三部分。

一、项目计划

1. 项目概况分析

与客户进行充分沟通,确定要翻译的任务范围、能够获得的参考资源(如以前翻译的旧版本、现有术语表、翻译记忆库等),以及目标读者的设定,其中目标读者的确定是至关重要的。传统的翻译服务首先要着眼于源文本的表面语言结构,其次或许会考虑目标受众。"信、达、雅"是评估翻译质量的铁标准。现代商业社会的语言服务则是以目标语言市场为中心,着重考虑的是翻译的目的、语境和受众沟通。一篇文本没有唯一正确的译文,而是针对不同的目标读者和预期用途存在不同的译文,所以必须要与客户就项目用途、目标读者、使用语境进行充分沟通。另外,客户已经拥有的项目相关语言资产是已被认可过的,是非常重要的参考资源,有时候无法从客户沟通中获得的信息反而能从旧的语言资产中获得。因此,开始项目前获得项目的相关信息和资源是非常关键的环节。

《新冠肺炎中医防治读本》项目要求项目经理在开始项目策划方案之前与客户(翻译任务委任方)进行深入沟通,明确该书英文版的发行市场和目标读者,清楚它的文本类型(见图 9-1),这对后续风格指南的制定以及具体翻译过程中的翻译决策起到至关重要的决定作用(见图 9-2)。因此,项目经理在获取相关信息后还需要和译员及审校人员也就此进行充分沟通。

2. 角色分工安排

翻译项目中最基础的三个角色是项目经理、译员和审校,如果客户有需求,还有

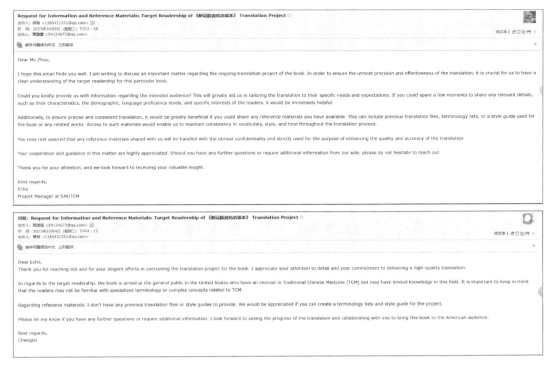

图9-1　2021级项目组询问客户目标读者以及参考资料的邮件往来

风格指南

文本定位：中医药科普读物（可复习外宣翻译课程的科普读物讲义）

中医药英文科普读物是广大海外读者了解中医药文化的重要窗口。科普读物属于普通科技文体，具有科学性、通俗性和文学性的特点，语篇正式度比专用科技文体低，用词平易、句式简单、多用修辞格（王国凤，2014：189-191）。为促进海外受众的理解和认知，达到良好的传播效果，科普读物译者需注重海外受众的信息需求和文化背景，借鉴西方英文科普读物的篇章和语言特征，在传递中医药文化内涵的前提下，运用目标受众熟悉的话语方式和表达方式适当进行变通翻译。

目标读者：喜欢中医药文化的外国读者（中医药知识储备不多）

风格及格式参考平行文本：Health Care in Eleventh Century China

图9-2　2021级项目组在其《风格指南》里明确文本定位和目标读者

可能加上排版人员、测试人员、技术人员等。要根据项目具体情况评估寻找适合的人员，并分配每个角色所需人员数量以及相应的工作内容。此案例中每组为五人，包含项目经理一人，译员两人，审校两人，按照字数相对平均的原则，分配了不同的章节翻译任务（见表9-1）。另外，为确保真实项目的翻译质量，还可以安排资深老师进行二审或三审。

表 9-1　2020 级项目组的角色分工安排表

项目	总字数	译员	交付时间	审校	交付时间	终审(教师)	交付时间
Part 1	1 280	同学 1	3 月 23 日	同学 4	3 月 24 日	教师 1	3 月 25 日
Part 2	1 307	同学 2	3 月 23 日	同学 3	3 月 24 日		
Part 3	1 366	同学 3	3 月 23 日	同学 2	3 月 24 日	教师 2	3 月 25 日
Part 4	1 536	同学 4	3 月 23 日	同学 1	3 月 24 日		

3. 时间节点安排

时间节点安排是项目经理的基础工作之一，可通过绘制各类计划进度表来实时跟踪和监控，并对项目节点进度进行检查和分析(见图 9-3 和图 9-4)。

ID	任务名称	人员	备注	开始时间	结束时间	持续时间	完成
1	文本清洗	单蕾		2022-03-18	2022-03-18	1.0 日	0.0%
2	⊟ 翻译风格指南			2022-03-18	2022-03-22	5.0 日	0.0%
	制定初稿	all		2022-03-18	2022-03-20	3.0 日	0.0%
	审定终稿	all		2022-03-21	2022-03-22	2.0 日	0.0%
3	⊟ 制作术语表			2022-03-18	2022-03-22	5.0 日	0.0%
	⊟ 单语术语表			2022-03-18	2022-03-19	2.0 日	0.0%
	提取术语	李冉、朱静洲、刘欣、蓝涵哲	共8页，按学号顺序2页/人	2022-03-18	2022-03-18	1.0 日	0.0%
	审定终稿	单蕾		2022-03-19	2022-03-19	1.0 日	0.0%
	⊟ 双语术语表			2022-03-20	2022-03-22	3.0 日	0.0%
	翻译术语	李冉、朱静洲、刘欣、蓝涵哲	按学号顺序 平均分配	2022-03-20	2022-03-21	2.0 日	0.0%
	审定术语	李冉、朱静洲、刘欣、蓝涵哲	译者 交叉审校	2022-03-22	2022-03-22	1.0 日	0.0%
4	翻译原文	李冉、朱静洲、刘欣、蓝涵哲	按学号顺序 平均分配	2022-03-23	2022-03-26	4.0 日	0.0%
5	审校译文	李冉、朱静洲、刘欣、蓝涵哲	译者 交叉审校	2022-03-27	2022-03-29	3.0 日	0.0%
6	排版交付	单蕾		2022-03-30	2022-03-30	1.0 日	0.0%

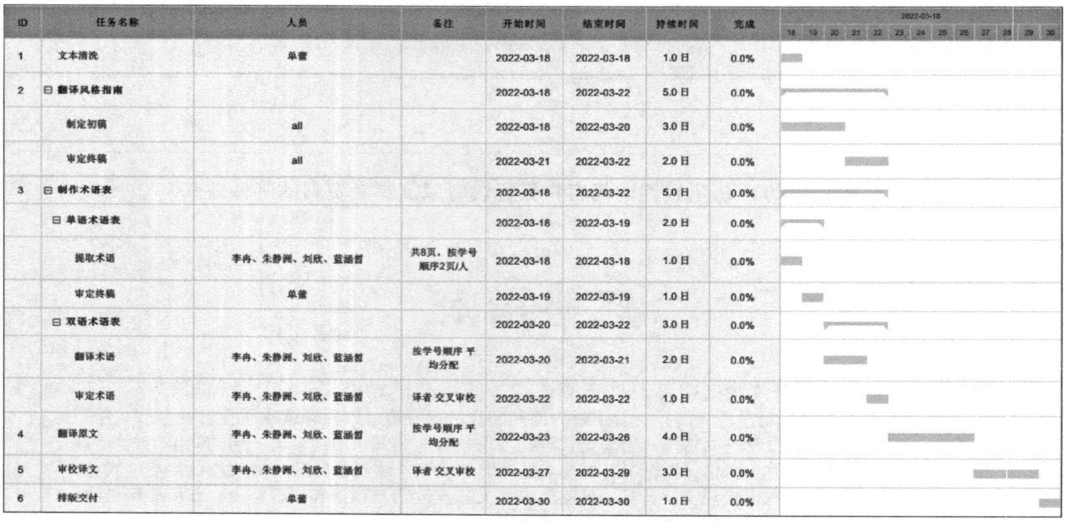

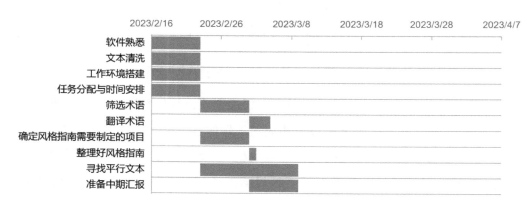

图 9-3　2020 级项目组的项目排期表

图 9-4　2021 级项目组的时间节点安排

4. 术语维护安排

由于术语是一个多人协作翻译项目开展的头号挑战,所以需要专门就术语库的创建和维护作出详细说明(见图9-5),并使用在线协作工具(如石墨文档)共同创建术语表(见图9-6)。

成员	术语提取并翻译+内容删减	翻译	审校
薛玲玲	01	01	04
刘萍萍	02	02	03
浦文怡	03	03	02
张晓晨	04	04	01

术语翻译优先参照世中联,不确定的讨论后处理
中药材 英文(拉丁语)

eg. 甘草：Liquorice Root (Radix Glycyrrhizae)

书名 英文(拼音)

eg. 《黄帝内经》：Huangdi's Internal Classic (Huangdi Neijing)

术语表样式：中文 英文 备注(解释如有)
术语提取规定
词频>2(见初始版本)
其余专业性词汇,如：
中医概念(疠气、瘟疫)
西医术语(病毒、治疗方式)
中药材：英文+拉丁语
方剂：英文+拼音(意群)
穴位(编码)
书名：《瘟疫论》
组织机构
头衔
传统度量单位(小写拼音)如：寸 cun 钱 qian 分 fen

图9-5　2021级项目组术语表创建计划

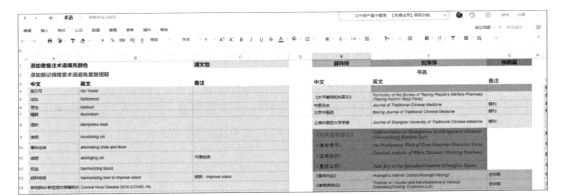

图9-6　2021级项目组利用石墨文档进行术语库创建和维护

5. 译审流程安排

通常在一个笔译项目的译审流程中有三个核心环节：翻译（Translation）、审校（Editing）、校对（Proofreading），审校偏向于审核校对文字层面的问题，而校对则偏向于总体上对格式、风格的调整。一个项目中还可能涉及多位译者和审校，甚至有行业专家审校的参与，那么如何合理分配人员、合理规划这三个环节将是项目成功执行与否的关键。一般在译员翻译后，由一般审校人员进行逐一文字校对的审校环节，也可称为一审；接着由资深审校或专家审校进行校对，即二审，通常关注点在译文专业度和文风、格式上；最后还可以由项目经理作最终的总体校对（见表9-1）。

6. 文件上传及命名方式

翻译项目经常涉及多个文件的操作，多人员的协作也会导致文件数量的倍数级增加，这就对项目经理的文件管理能力提出了更高的要求。文件管理的重点是文件夹和文件命名以及文件分类。清晰、简洁和一致的命名规则有助于确保文件的有效管理和组织，并提高项目的效率和可追溯性。通常文件夹或文件命名需要包含项目名称、语言对（原文语言到目标语言）、文件类型、日期等。例如："项目名称_源语言-目标语言_文件类型_日期"。日期可以区分多个版本的文件。

7. 译员培训会

对译员传达以上重要信息，并根据译员情况进行相关的软件熟悉或技术培训。做好会议纪要。

二、文件预处理

预处理主要是对相关翻译文档、术语表、历史文件、参考资料等做翻译前的处理工作，为之后能够在 CAT 软件内成功创建项目做准备，具体包括以下内容。

1. 文字识别

如果原文是不可编辑版的 PDF，需要运用 OCR 软件进行光学文字识别。通常可以使用 Abbyy Finereader 或 Adobe Acrobat 软件进行文字识别和清洁。

2. 文本拆分

因为是基于单机版的计算机辅助翻译协作，所以需要在导入 CAT 工具前根据译员的任务分配对原文进行拆分。拆分文件可直接在 Office Word 中进行，并分别导入 CAT 软件的翻译项目中。

3. 创建 CAT 可用的双语术语库

任何一门专业学科都存在着大量的专业术语，专业术语是学科的理论基础，往往只有该专业领域的人士才能充分理解和掌握。术语是翻译人员在翻译专业类材料时碰到的最难以逾越的障碍,因为术语翻译得是否专业地道直接决定了这篇翻译像不像"业内人士说的话"。而中医学作为一门历史悠久、理论丰富的学科,术语众多且繁杂,翻译中医类相关材料的最大难点之一当然也是术语。现代化的翻译可以通过各类术语软件实现术语的数字化管理,根据专业领域收集术语及其翻译以及使用规则录入数据库中。这样的数据库可以实现实时搜索查找,大大提高译员翻译专业领域材料的专业度。术语库管理一般要在译前就准备好,创建为双语术语库并导入 CAT工具中,这样在译中才能实时获取术语的翻译。

术语在现代化翻译中的另一个重要意义是保持翻译的一致性,这是企业在全球化过程中进行语言资产管理的重要环节。如前文所述,现代语言服务行业大多涉及多平台、多模态、多文本、结构化的翻译项目,翻译的内容量成倍增长,参与翻译项目的人员也越来越多,这个时候,一致性的问题就尤为突出。术语管理做得越完善,术语一致性就越好,翻译质量也越高。前文中关于译前项目计划的术语创建维护(见图9-5)就展示了项目经理在译前计划阶段对术语的创建和维护进行的总体规划安排。《新冠肺炎中医防治读本》是一本中医科普类读本,其内容较浅显易懂,但涉及多个中医分支学科,比如中药术语、方剂术语、功法术语、穴位术语、典籍书名等。译前创建术语库并导入 CAT 工具,才能实现基于单机版软件的翻译项目协作,并有效解决协作过程中的术语一致性问题。

译前术语库的创建目前来说自动化程度不高,许多工作仍需人工完成,一般分为术语提取(网络工具根据词频提取以及人工提取)(见图9-7和图9-8)、术语筛选(人工界定术语、分类术语)、术语翻译(可根据项目情况参考现有官方或认可度高的中医术语翻译,比如 WHO 术语翻译、世中联中医术语翻译等)(见图9-5中利用石墨文档在线协作平台实现术语筛选和术语翻译的协作),最后形成一份项目专用的术语表,然后利用 CAT 工具创建术语库(见图9-9),最后在 CAT 中创建项目时可同时导入术语库,使得多个译员在同时翻译时还能够保持术语翻译的一致性和文风的统一(王华树,2016:81)。

4. 创建 CAT 可用的翻译记忆库

此处的翻译记忆库包括两大类:一类是新建的项目翻译记忆库,即要用于此次翻译项目的空翻译记忆库,在翻译的过程中不断填充该记忆库。另一类是已经存有历史数据的翻译记忆库,其中的数据可以是以前翻译的旧版本的译文。如果没有,也可以不添加。

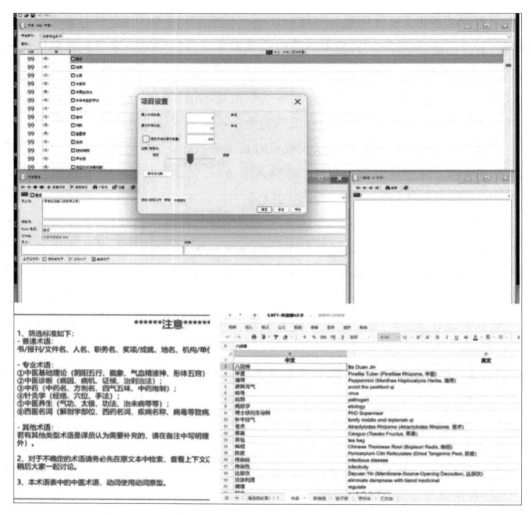

图 9 - 7 2021 级项目组利用 SDL MultiTerm Extract 提取术语

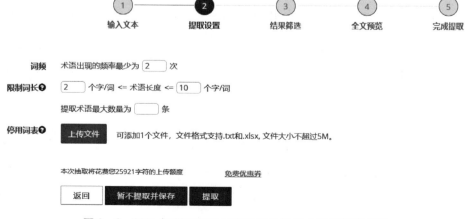

图 9 - 8 2021 级项目组利用在线平台语帆术语宝提取术语

	A	B
1	中文	英文
2	疏风	disperse wind
3	拇指	thumb
4	上海	Shanghai
5	驱邪	eliminate pathogenic factors
6	防疫	epidemic prevention
7	三钱	9.375 g
8	颗粒	Granule
9	机体	the body
10	麻黄	Ephedra (Ephedrae Herba, 麻黄)
11	二分或三分	0.625 g or 0.9375 g
12	胸部影像学	chest imaging
13	防风通圣丸	Fangfeng Tongsheng Pills
14	手掌大鱼际	thenar region
15	安宫牛黄丸	Angong Niuhuang Pills
16	荆防败毒散	Jing Fang Baidu San (Fineleaf Schizonepeta Herb and Divaricate Saposhnikovia Root Baidu Powder, 荆防败毒散)
17	开上焦肺气	ventilate the Lung qi of the Upper jiao
18	中医治疗篇	Treatment with TCM
19	恢复调护篇	Recovery with TCM
20	固本预防篇	Prevention with TCM
21	石菖蒲	Grassleaf Sweetflag Rhizome (Acori Tatarinowii Rhizoma, 石菖蒲)
22	白茅根	Lalang Grass Rhizome (Imperatae Rhizoma, Baimaogen, 白茅根)
23	影像学	chest imaging
24	杨爱东	YANG Aidong
25	重症期	critical stage

图 9－9　2021 级项目组制作的术语表截图

三、译前准备

1. 平行文本检索

研究平行文本的语言特点和行文风格是译员能够在短时间内提高译文的可读性和影响力的有效方法。不管是外宣文本中的信息型文本、表情型文本还是操作型文本，根据其要实现的交际目的和面对的目标读者的不同，都应选择相应类型的平行文本作为翻译参考。另外，当译入语是译者的非母语时，平行文本能起到的作用更为明显。中医药翻译多为中文译为其他语言，因此译入语是译者的非母语的情况居多，那么译者可以在译前搜索相同或类似交际目的的中医相关平行文本，学习母语者的地道表达方式和行文规范，提高译文的可接受性。平行文本也是后续创建风格指南的重要指导性参考文件之一。

《新冠肺炎中医防治读本》翻译项目的目标读者是对中医感兴趣但相关知识储备有限的美国普通民众。文体为外宣科普读物。项目经理、译员、审校人员搜索了网络上英文版本的中医科普以及医学科普类文章进行研读分析，也可根据新冠肺炎预防和治疗这一主题搜索类似的西医或其他中医类版本作为参考。

2020 级项目组参考的平行文本为中英版《新冠肺炎防治手册(标准版)》、中英版《新型冠状病毒感染的肺炎公众防护指南》和英文版 *COVID-19 from Traditional*

Chinese Medicine Perspective。2021 级项目组参考的则是同为医学科普类的文本 *Health Care in Eleventh-Century China*。平行文本不管是在翻译策略的选择上,还是在文本呈现格式上都有着重要的参考意义。比如,《新冠肺炎中医防治读本》中有较多中医相关类术语,例如中药名、方剂名、中医类书籍名称、穴位名等,对于这类术语的翻译,如果要同时提供中文和拼音,那么应该以怎样的格式呈现才更符合目标市场的科普类文章的要求? 2021 级项目组通过翻看 *Health Care in Eleventh-Century China* 找到了类似的书写格式:即英文译文后加括号,括号内先拼音,后中文(见图 9 - 10),因此对于中医类书籍名称的翻译也采用了同样的格式(见图 9 - 11)。

The Diversity of Health Care   3

studying the conventional classics, they learned their trade by memorizing the written classics of their field, and—mostly but not always—learning current methods as disciples or apprentices. They competed with members of hereditary medical families, who passed down proprietary therapies. These retainers remained the majority of therapists to the gentry and others who could afford them. By the Song period, many of that group had learned to read and write, at least well enough to keep records. Some were indistinguishable from the literate physicians.[4]

Since there was no organization to police qualifications, anyone could call himself a doctor (*yisheng* 醫生 or *yi* 醫). Many with scantier educations cultivated a clientèle further down the social scale. Further still down the scale, people with more limited skills tended to present themselves as "therapists (*yishi* 醫士 or *yigong* 醫工)" rather than "physicians." Where the boundary lay was merely a matter for curer and patient to agree on. There was also an indistinct genre of itinerant curers, called "neighborhood therapists (*lüyan yigong* 閭閻醫工)" "doctors of the grassy marshes (*caoze yi* 草澤醫)," "bell-ringing doctors (*lingyi* 鈴醫)," and by other names.[5]

图 9 - 10 平行文本 *Health Care in Eleventh-Century China*

Puji Xiaodu Yin (Universal Relief Decoction for Disinfection, 普济消毒饮)

Source: *Dong Yuan Trying Efficacy of Formulas (Dongyuan Shixiao Fang, 东垣试效方)* written by Li Gao

Formulation: Baical Skullcap Root (Scutellaeiae Radix, 黄芩) (processed by wine) and Golden Thread (Coptidis Rhizoma, 黄连) 15.625 g respectively; Pericarpium Citri Reticulatae (Dried Tangerine Peel, 陈皮), Liquorice Root (Radix Glycyrrhizae, 甘草) (raw), Figwort Root (Scrophulariae Radix, 玄参), Chinese Thorowax Root (Bupleuri Radix, 柴胡) and Platycodon Root (Radix Platycodonis, 桔梗) 6.25 g respectively; Forsythia (Forsythia Suspensa, 连翘), Indigowoad Root (Isatidis Radix, 板蓝根), Puff Ball (Lasiosphaera Seu Calvatia, 马勃), Great Burdock Achene (Arctii Fructus, 牛蒡子) and Peppermint (Menthae Haplocalycis Herba, 薄荷) 3.125g respectively; Stiff Silkworm (Bombys Batryticatus, 僵蚕) and Largetrifoliolious Bugbane Rhizome (Cimicifugae Rhizoma, 升麻) 0.014 g respectively

图 9 - 11 《新冠防治读本》中对于中医类书籍名称的翻译

2. 创建风格指南

团队协作的方式可能会带来不同的文字表达风格、不同的术语翻译策略、不同的行文格式规范。为了让所有内容保持高度的一致性和明确性,就需要一份指导性的文件来规范所有参与人员(主要是译员和审校人员)的翻译风格。风格指南一般包括以下几个部分(凯瑞·J. 以恩、埃琳娜·S. 邓恩,2017：110)：

- 项目概览：描述项目的目标受众和交际目的。
- 写作风格：概述行文风格特点。
- 一般格式：规定如动词时态、引用拼写、标点符号、字体、字号、标题大小写、本地化(如当地货币、时间、地址)等一般性的格式,可参考微软等出版的技术出版风格指南。
- 术语格式：规定专业术语的最佳表述方式,比如《新冠肺炎中医防治读本》里中药和方剂等的翻译中,英文译文、拉丁文、拼音、中文等应该保留哪几个,以何种顺序出现。
- 注意事项示例：可以提供能够参考的所有规则的真实示例,明确什么样的是"该做"的,什么样的是"不该做"的。重点指出什么是需要避免的。

风格指南一般可以由客户或语言专家提供,也可以由项目经理、译员和审校人员在译前通读原文、咨询客户以及参考网络资料,共同商讨撰写本次项目的风格指南(见图 9-12 和图 9-13)。风格指南同时也是动态的,在译中可以更新,但需要项目经理设置好更新的方式,以免新旧版本发生错乱。

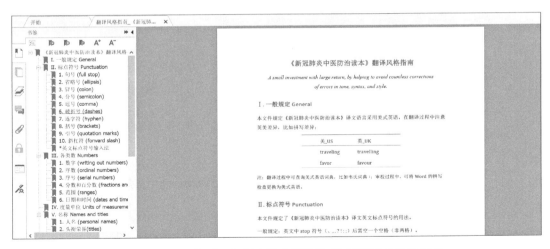

图 9-12　2020 级项目组制定的 8 项规定、32 项细则的风格指南

3. 创建 CAT 翻译项目

项目经理把在预处理环节内准备好的待译文档、术语库、翻译记忆库(如有)、参考资料等导入 CAT 创建翻译项目。

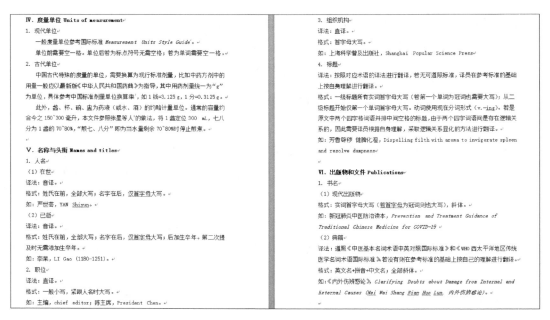

图 9 - 13　2021 级项目组的风格指南(部分)

4. 文档分析

文档分析包括文件字数分析、文档重复率计算。

5. 通过 CAT 工具向译员发包

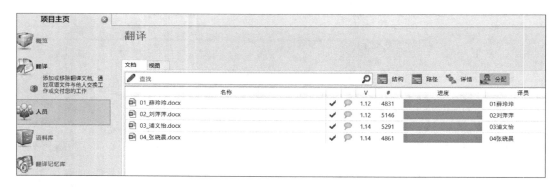

图 9 - 14　2021 级项目组在计算机辅助翻译软件 memoQ 中任务发包

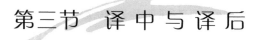

第三节　译中与译后

译中主要由项目经理负责调节翻译进度,组织译稿审校,并最终排版定稿。因此,此阶段主要包括项目执行的翻译、一审、二审、排版定稿,以及项目的进度控制和质量保证。由于这是教学与真实项目实践相结合的项目教学活动,因此这一阶段的人员流程为项目经理—译员—学生一审—教师二审—项目经理,四者之间形成闭环关系。

译后主要是译文提交和收尾工作,将最终译文根据客户要求提交给客户后,项目组所有成员进行项目反思和经验分享,并对项目实践过程中所产生的语言资产进行整理和归档。教师可布置学生撰写项目总结报告,进行技术操作和翻译实践上的反思,并在项目组内互相分享讨论。语言资产的整理和归档主要由项目经理操作,以便为下一个翻译项目提供参考文件。

一、翻译

译员在 CAT 工具中导入项目经理发来的项目文件包,并在软件内进行翻译,根据项目经理制定的进度安排,督促协调译员完成各自的翻译任务。在译前项目计划的项目概况分析中,项目经理通过和客户的沟通而获得了关于目标读者的信息,并且将这个关键信息写到风格指南的醒目位置,让译者和审校人员对所进行的翻译项目的文本类型、目标读者都有充分理解。因此,在具体的翻译时,这一理解应贯彻整个翻译过程,并且但凡遇到翻译策略选择问题时,都是至关重要的考虑因素。

以下是 2021 级项目组三位同学的课后总结的部分内容摘录,涉及他们作为译员在《新冠肺炎中医防治读本》翻译项目中碰到需要选择不同译法时,会如何根据文本类型和目标读者做出适合的翻译策略选择。

摘录 1:

在译前各项工作中应该将读者需求和客户要求考虑在内,这一意识是我们大家普遍缺乏的。在真实的翻译项目中,作为乙方工作者,甲方的要求我们必须听取,但是对于何类内容需要听取客户意见,这一点我们还是要明确的。因为甲方可能对于过于专业性的翻译问题了解不深,所以我们不应向客户提过于专业的问题。可以就文章整体风格等问题咨询客户。就读者意识来说,我认为在我们组的翻译中也有所体现。例如,我们将文中的古代度量单位("钱"和"两"等)统一为现代度量单位"g",这其实就是一种读者意识的体现,采用现代度量单位有利于外国读者的理解。

摘录 2:

翻译中要充分考虑到文体和受众,这次的新冠防治手册为科普读物,所以在翻译中我也尽量保证语句简洁、通俗、易懂,对一些冗余的、不必要的描述进行适当的删减省译,保证文本的流畅性和易读性。例如在翻译"大便无力"一词时,"大便、排便"一词主要的翻译有 defecation 和 bowel movement,通过 COCA 语料库词频查询,bowel movement 使用频率更高。鉴于该文为科普文,用词也需更为简单,通俗易懂,故而最终选用 bowel movement。

摘录3:

虽然文本属于科普类文本,但是由于中医语料内涵丰富,对译者的背景知识也有一定的要求。在处理术语规范化的问题上,应该不断搜索和查阅(必要时可以考虑咨询专业人士),尤其是某些官方标准,例如世中联术语、WHO 术语、《黄帝内经》译本等等。遇到理解问题时,应该积极讨论,广泛搜索。在翻译策略选择的问题上,应从受众的角度出发,采取多元化的翻译策略,例如节译、改译、编译、译写等等,关注受众的信息需求和文化背景,对原文稿件进行适当加工和处理,借鉴西方英文科普读物的篇章和语言特征,在传递中医药文化内涵的前提下,运用目标受众熟悉的话语方式和表达方式适当进行变通翻译。

二、审校

项目经理在确保译稿信息完整、文风恰当、格式正确的情况下分发至学生一审进行审校,一审完成后在 CAT 工具内做一般 QA(Quality Assurance,质量保证)后发送至教师二审进行最终审稿。项目经理在翻译和审校的过程中需要进行调整术语库的更新工作。另外,在教师的指导下,对于译者和审校人员提出的任何相关问题提供支持,处理客户咨询和反馈等,提升翻译的专业性和质量,积累实践经验。

三、排版定稿

项目经理获得最终译稿后,进行最终 QA,检查翻译一致性、术语一致性、是否违背风格指南的规定等,然后导出译文,视客户实际需求进行图、表、文等多样文本类型和文字格式的排版工作。

四、进度控制和质量保证

这一环节的操作融合在译中部分前三个环节内进行。

五、译后语言资产维护

在整个项目操作过程中所产生的包括但不限于术语库、风格指南、翻译记忆库(CAT 工具将原文和译文通过——对应的句对方式进行保存的文件)等都可以作为下一次类似任务的参考文件。所以项目经理可以在项目结束后进行整理归类保存。不管是充当项目中的哪种角色,都可以在项目完成后,积极撰写项目总结,概括经验,归纳学到的知识,这对以后其他项目的开展是非常有益的。

第四节　翻译练习与任务

一、翻译任务

假设你目前是一名翻译或翻译项目经理,某个出版社客户希望你能帮忙翻译或组织翻译一本中医类书籍《思考中医》,请利用计算机辅助翻译软件,以小组协作的方式将书籍《思考中医》翻译为英文版本。要求能够切合目标语言市场、制定完整高效的多人协作流程、创建专业可用的术语库,使语言质量达到出版水平,格式尽量与原文保持一致。

1. 任务说明

1)原文名称:《思考中医》

2)出版信息:

作者:刘力红

出版社:广西师范大学出版社

*出版时间:*2003 年 6 月

ISBN:9787563339198

3)原文语言:简体中文

4)原文格式:PDF

5)目标语言:美式英语

6)项目周期:21 天

2. 具体要求

1)学员分组:共分 2 组(练习组和项目组),5 人/组

2)角色分工:项目经理、译员、审校

3)翻译软件:memoQ 软件

4)项目经理:

• 设计和撰写翻译协作方案(包括任务分析、角色分工、流程安排、时间安排等)

- 创建项目
- 分配任务
- 监督进度
- 回收任务
- 合成译文
- 导出译文
- 撰写项目总结与反思、提交所有要求的项目文件

5）**译员审校：**

- 接收任务
- 完成翻译或审校工作
- 交付任务
- 软件翻译或审校功能应用
- 问题解决

6）**交付要求：**

- 翻译协作方案（成员分工流程及时间节点表、风格指南、术语表）
- 每个小组总的项目文件+协作过程文件+个人项目文件+个人总结
- 排版后的译文文件（Word 和 PDF 各一份）

3. 任务分解与操作

- **项目管理任务**（撰写项目方案及角色分工、准备术语库、创建项目、统计工作量、分配任务、监督进度、合成并交付译文）
- **文本翻译任务**（接受任务、软件翻译功能应用、翻译资源共享、实时 QA 处理、翻译问题解决、提交任务）
- **文本审校任务**（接受任务、自定义 QA 参数、QA 问题处理、人工审校、QA 报告）
- **技术支持任务**（协助安装翻译软件、处理文本格式、提取术语、提取重复句段、译文排版、项目进行过程中各种技术问题的解决）

二、扩展阅读

［1］王华树. 翻译技术实践［M］. 北京：外文出版社,2016.

［2］凯瑞·J. 邓恩,埃琳娜·S. 邓恩. 翻译与本地化项目管理［M］. 王华树,于艳玲,译. 北京：知识产权出版社,2017.

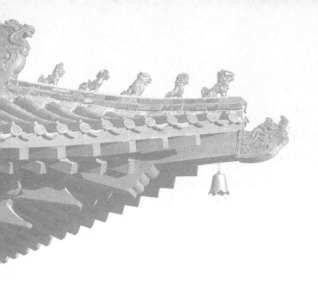

参考文献

［1］Genette, G. *Paratexts: Thresholds of Interpretation* [M]. (Tr. by Lewin J E; forwarded by Macksey R). Cambridge: Cambridge University Press, 1997.

［2］Hartmann, R. R. K. *Contrastive Textology: Comparative Discourse Analysis in Applied Linguistics*[M]. Heidelberg: Julius Groos Verlag, 1980.

［3］Lefevere, A. *Translation, Rewriting and the Manipulation of Literary Fame*[M]. London: Routledge, 1992.

［4］Munday, J. *Introducing Translation Studies: Theories and Applications* [M]. London/New York: Routledge, 2001.

［5］Nord, C. *Translating as a Purposeful Activity: Functional Approaches Explained* [M]. Shanghai: Shanghai Foreign Language Education Press, 2001.

［6］Nord, C. *Text Analysis in Translation: Theory, Methodology, and Didactic Application of a Model for Translation-oriented Text Analysis*[M]. Amsterdam and Atlanta, GA: Rodopi, 1991; Beijing: Foreign Language Teaching and Research Press, 2005.

［7］Nord, C. Looking for Help in the Translation Process—The Role of Auxiliary Texts in Translator Training and Translation Practice[J]. 中国翻译, 2007(1): 17 – 26.

［8］Reiss, K. *Text Types, Translation Types and Translation Assessment*[A]. (Tr. by Chesterman A). In Chesterman A (ed.). 1977/1989: 105 – 115.

［9］Reiss, K. *Type, Kind and Individuality of Text: Decision Making in Translation* [A]. (Tr. by S. Kitron). In Venuti L. ed. *The Translation Studies Reader*[C].

London / New York: Routledge, 1971/2000: 160 - 171.

[10] Swales, J. *Genre Analysis: English in Academic and Research Settings* [M]. Cambridge: Cambridge University Press, 1990.

[11] Swales, J. & Feak, C. *Academic Writing for Graduate Students: Essential Tasks and Skills*[M]. Ann Arbor: University of Michigan Press, 2012.

[12] Vermeer, H. J. Skopos and Commission in Translational Action[A]. In Chesterman A ed. *Readings in Translation Theory*[C]. Finland: Oy Finn Lectura Ab, 1989.

[13] Vermette, P. Four fatal flaws: Avoiding the common mistakes of novice users of cooperative learning[J]. *The High School Journal*, 1994, 77(3): 255 - 260.

[14] 爱泼斯坦,林戊荪,沈苏儒.呼吁重视对外宣传中的外语工作[J].中国翻译, 2000(6): 2 - 4.

[15] 曹志建.功能主义视角下的法律外宣文本翻译[M].广州：暨南大学出版社, 2016.

[16] 陈德兴,张玉萍,徐丽莉,等.神农本草经[M].福州：福建科学技术出版社, 2012.

[17] 陈戍国.周礼[M].长沙：岳麓书社,1989.

[18] 陈小慰.对德国翻译功能目的论的修辞反思[J].外语研究,2012(1): 91 - 95.

[19] 陈小慰.译有所依——汉英对比与翻译研究新路径[M].厦门：厦门大学出版社,2017.

[20] 戴宗显,吕和发.公示语汉英翻译研究——以2012年奥运会主办城市伦敦为例[J].中国翻译,2005,26(6): 38 - 42.

[21] 丁衡祁.努力完善城市公示语 逐步确定参照性译文[J].中国翻译,2006,27(6): 12 - 16.

[22] 都立澜,朱建平,洪梅.中医药名词术语英译策略与方法辨析及体系初步构建[J].中华中医药杂志,2020,35(6): 2838 - 2841.

[23] 段连城.对外传播学初探[M].北京：五洲传播出版社,2004.

[24] 方梦之.文类细化之于翻译培训、翻译策略——拓展应用翻译研究的领域(之二)[J].上海翻译,2017(3): 3 - 8+93.

[25] 方梦之,毛忠明.英汉—汉英应用翻译综合教程[M].上海：上海外语教育出版社,2018.

[26] 冯正斌,刘振清.新冠肺炎疫情防控外宣话语战争隐喻英译探赜——以《抗击新

冠肺炎疫情的中国行动》白皮书为例[J].渭南师范学院学报,2022,37(1):68-73.

[27] 高芸.中西医英语科研论文语篇互动性对比研究——基于 SCI 期刊论文的语料库分析[J].外语电化教学,2018(2):78-83.

[28] 高芸.中医翻译叙事能力培养的教学研究[J].中医教育,2020,39(4):65-68.

[29] 高芸.中医外宣翻译理论与教学实践[M].上海:上海交通大学出版社,2023.

[30] 胡洁.建构视角下的外宣翻译研究[D].上海:上海外国语大学,2010.

[31] 胡珍铭,王湘玲.评教整合的翻译教学模式构建与实践——以培养文本分析能力为导向[J].外语界,2018,189(6):79-86.

[32] 黄友义.坚持"外宣三贴近"原则,处理好外宣翻译中的难点问题[J].中国翻译,2004,25(6):27-28.

[33] 贾树枚解读.中国故事 国际表达——赵启正新闻传播案例[M].上海:上海人民出版社,2018.

[34] 杰里米·芒迪.翻译学导论:理论与应用[M].李德凤,等,译.北京:外语教学与研究出版社,2014.

[35] 凯瑞·J. 邓恩,埃琳娜·S. 邓恩.翻译与本地化项目管理[M].王华树,于艳玲,译.北京:知识产权出版社,2017.

[36] 李长栓.非文学翻译理论与实践[M].北京:中国对外翻译出版公司,2004.

[37] 李德超,王克非.平行文本比较模式与旅游文本的英译[J].中国翻译,2009(4):54-58.

[38] 李运兴.语篇翻译引论[M].北京:中国对外翻译出版公司,2001.

[39] 李照国.中医英语翻译技巧[M].北京:人民卫生出版社,1997.

[40] 李照国.中医名词术语英译国际标准化新进展——从世界卫生组织传统医学国际分类东京会议谈起[J].中西医结合学报,2011,9(1):113-115.

[41] 李照国.中医英语翻译研究[M].上海:上海三联书店,2013.

[42] 李照国.中医基本名词术语英译研究[M].西安:世界图书出版西安有限公司,2017.

[43] 廖七一.当代西方翻译理论探索[M].南京:译林出版社,2000.

[44] 刘季春.实用翻译教程(第三版)[M].广州:中山大学出版社,2016.

[45] 刘明,汪顺,范琳琳,等.中药药品英文说明书撰写的研究综述与今后研究方向的探讨[J].中医药导报,2016,22(21):117-125.

［46］卢小军.国家形象与外宣翻译策略研究［M］.北京：外语教学与研究出版社，
2015.

［47］罗海燕，邓海静.文本类型理论指导下的中医外宣资料英译［J］.中国中医基础
医学杂志，2017(4)：567－569.

［48］罗茜.评价系统视角下中医形象构建的话语策略研究——以《中国的中医药》白
皮书英译本为例［J］.中医文献杂志，2019,37(6)：32－36.

［49］马有度.奇妙中医药——家庭保健顾问［M］.北京：人民卫生出版社，2009.

［50］梅美莲，杨仙菊.含 No 和 Only 的英语公示语研究［J］.西安外国语大学学报，
2013,21(4)：58－61.

［51］牛新生.从感召功能看汉语公示语英译——以宁波城市公示语为例［J］.中国翻
译，2007(2)：63－67.

［52］任文.新时代语境下翻译人才培养模式再探究：问题与出路［J］.当代外语研
究，2018(6)：92－98.

［53］宋世豪，童林，朱文晓.浅析目的论视域下中医院公示语英译原则——以郑州 3
所中医院为例［J］.中国校外教育，2018(11)：95－96.

［54］孙小春.汉语公示语英文译写的语用阐释［J］.上海翻译，2020(3)：40－44.

［55］孙中有.理解当代中国：汉英翻译教程［M］.北京：外语教学与研究出版社，
2022.

［56］谭益兰.从语篇分析角度研究西藏旅游景点公示语汉英语篇翻译［J］.西藏大学
学报(社会科学版)，2013,28(4)：57－64.

［57］涂雯.文本类型理论指导下的中成药说明书功能与主治英译研究［D］.北京：北
京中医药大学，2018.

［58］王畅，杨玉晨.生态翻译学视角下 TCM 医院公示语英译研究［J］.上海翻译，
2018(4)：39－43.

［59］王笃勤.英语教学策略论［M］.北京：外语教学与研究出版社，2002.

［60］王国凤.新编英汉翻译实用教程［M］.浙江：浙江大学出版社，2014.

［61］王华树.翻译技术实践［M］.北京：外文出版社，2016.

［62］王宁.翻译与国家形象的建构及海外传播［J］.外语教学，2018,39(5)：1－6.

［63］王树槐.翻译教学论［M］.上海：上海外语教育出版社，2013.

［64］王雪玉.论文摘要英译中的作者身份建构［J］.现代语文，2016(8)：136－140.

［65］魏迺杰(Nigel Wiseman).英汉·汉英中医词典［M］.长沙：湖南科学技术出版

社,1996.

[66] 文师吾,谢日华.SCI 医学英文论文的撰写与发表[M].北京:人民卫生出版社,2012.

[67] 夏天.平行文本运用与汉英翻译教学"去技巧化"[J].外语电化教学,2015(4):17－22.

[68] 肖琼.中成药说明书中功效术语的生态化翻译研究[J].郑州航空工业管理学院学报(社会科学版),2014,33(6):100－103.

[69] 谢丹.变译在公示语汉英翻译中的应用[M].成都:西南交通大学出版社,2017.

[70] 谢天振.译介学:理念创新与学术前景[J].外语学刊,2019,209(4):95－102.

[71] 辛红娟,严文钏.关联理论视角下的隐喻翻译研究——以《抗击新冠肺炎疫情的中国行动》英译为例[J].宁波大学学报(人文科学版),2022,35(4):79－84.

[72] 熊兵.基于英汉双语平行语料库的翻译教学模式研究[J].外语界,2015(4):2－10.

[73] 徐铫伟,周领顺.翻译教学、实践和研究中的"求真"与"务实"——周领顺教授访谈录[J].语言教育,2020,8(3):2－7+13.

[74] 杨冬青.纽马克翻译理论指导下的白皮书汉译英[J].西南农业大学学报(社会科学版),2013,11(6):112－115.

[75] 杨丰宁.英汉语言比较与翻译[M].天津:天津大学出版社,2006.

[76] 叶朗,朱良志.中国文化读本[M].北京:外语教学与研究出版社,2016.

[77] 余环,邓凌云.中国文化"走出去"背景下的职业译者能力研究[J].上海翻译,2019(5):40－45.

[78] 曾剑平.外宣翻译的中国特色与话语融通[J].江西社会科学,2018,38(10):239－245.

[79] 张健.报刊语言翻译[M].北京:高等教育出版社,2008.

[80] 张健.全球化语境下的外宣翻译"变通"策略刍议[J].外国语言文学,2013a,30(1):19－27+43+72.

[81] 张健.外宣翻译导论[M].北京:国防工业出版社,2013b.

[82] 张健.新闻英语文体与范文评析[M].上海:上海外语教育出版社,2016.

[83] 张健,许天虎.企业简介英译若干问题探讨[J].上海翻译,2019(6):36－40+28.

［84］张美芳.翻译中的超文本成分：以新闻翻译为例［J］.中国翻译,2011(2)：50－55.

［85］张美芳.文本类型、翻译目的及翻译策略［J］.上海翻译,2013(4)：5－10.

［86］张小萌,李芳.多模态视域下英国公示语特征研究——以新冠疫情下英国多层级公示语为例［J］.现代语言学,2022,10(5)：1046－1053.

［87］赵家明.政府文献翻译的话语实践研究——以中美经贸磋商白皮书英译和传播为例［D］.吉林大学,2022.

［88］郑玲.中医英语译写教程［M］.北京：中医古籍出版社,2013.